Totally Bound Publishing titles from these authors:

By Cheryl Dragon

Fantasy Castle
Kat's Karma

I0663232

Paid Holiday
One Weekend
Keeping It Interesting
A Firm Hand

Anthologies:
Tied to the Billionaire: Devoted to Him

By Megan Slayer

Permanent
Vaulting

OUT OF BOUNDS ANTHOLOGY

MAKING THE PASS
CHERYL DRAGON

CROSSING THE LINE
MEGAN SLAYER

IN THE RED ZONE
STEPHANIE BURKE

Out of Bounds Anthology
ISBN # 978-1-78184-644-5
Making the Pass ©Copyright Cheryl Dragon 2013
Crossing the Line ©Copyright Megan Slayer 2013
In the Red Zone ©Copyright Stephanie Burke 2013
Cover Art by Posh Gosh ©Copyright May 2013
Interior text design by Claire Siemaszkiewicz
Totally Bound Publishing

Published in 2013 by Totally Bound Publishing, Newland House, The Point, Weaver Road, Lincoln, LN6 3QN, United Kingdom.

Totally Bound Publishing is an imprint of Total-E-Ntwined Limited.

MAKING THE PASS

Cheryl Dragon

Dedication

For Megan Slayer, who made the antho happen!

Chapter One

Aiden Brewer kept his eye on the ball and the field. The last summer wind blew over his arms as the evening brought cooler temps to the New England football field. It was just a practice so the stands were empty and after he'd bruised his ribs in the last game, Aiden wasn't pushing too hard. Looking over at Jack Allman eased the pain with a jolt of lust. A field full of hot men and Aiden had to want the one who showed no real interest. They were friends but not really that close.

It made Aiden nuts. Especially when he had to target Jack with the ball. The wide receiver had good hands and fast feet. He also had sexy boy-next-door looks on an athletically muscled body with buzzed reddish brown hair. His chest hair tempted Aiden even more. Those deep brown eyes of his never missed a thing in the locker room.

Aiden had to lead and shook off the fantasy of tackling Jack naked. Facing the same direction, Jack squatted a few feet away. Aiden was always aware of where Jack was since passing the football to Jack was

Aiden's job. As he reached for the ball, Aiden swore Jack was looking at him. .

Ignoring Jack, Aiden took off and ran the play. He found Jack down the field and hurled the ball with precision. His ribs screamed and Aiden held his side. His teammates didn't tackle him and Paul came over. Aiden watched Jack's strong body power down the field and make a touchdown. His ass looked so good in that uniform, Aiden wondered if he'd ever get over the friend who seemed oblivious.

"You okay?" Paul asked.

"Just the ribs. Damn, still sore." He tried to shake it off.

"You're thirty. You're not going to bounce back like those wild twenties anymore." Paul patted him on the back.

"I just didn't want to sit it out." Aiden shrugged.

"Why not? You won't turn rusty in a week." Despite Paul being a good friend, Aiden didn't want to hear it.

Aiden nodded to the other end of the field. "Jack as usual. Being a dick."

"He said something?" Paul asked.

"In the locker room. He's two years older but no sympathy." Aiden knew Jack's job was more physical. The advantage of having more muscle was all with Jack, at least for muscle and power. The perfect throws were Aiden. The engineer had to hit his mark.

"You should just freak him out. Kiss him or something. I bet that'd solve a lot of problems," Paul teased.

Aiden shook his head. "I'm not being the butt of more of his jokes. The guy has it in for me."

"Not how you think," Paul said.

That train of thought would only get Aiden into trouble. Jack could take the teasing if Aiden chose to dish it back.

The assistant coach blew his whistle and the team headed in. "Good job. Hit the showers. Aiden, don't push it next practice. Rest the ribs so you're good for the game. Sitting out one won't kill you."

"Sure." Aiden pulled off his helmet.

"But hit the gym so you stay loose." Jack grinned as they walked towards the showers.

"You're the coach now too? Why don't you just pass yourself the ball?" Aiden shot back.

The team laughed and headed for the showers. Aiden knew his banter with Jack was expected. The duo always delivered. He found Jack and Jack somehow managed to outrun the tight end and nab the pass. They were connected and the team counted on them. Plenty of guys gave them crap about being a couple. Practising at home and on the side – Aiden wished!

He was last in the steam-filled college locker room. The facilities were updated and well-maintained. He sat on the extra-wide bench down the middle of the rows of lockers. There was no rush. As annoying as Jack could be, Aiden hated leaving the games and practices.

Paul helped him get the pads off to spare his ribs. When the material cleared his head, Aiden caught Jack watching. The man was nuts! Running his mouth then acting jealous. Paul was a friend and had eyes for that kicker on the Griffins' rival team. Aiden hated to turn the tables of teasing on Paul, but it'd work.

Plus that topic was the one source of fun Jack would jump on immediately and side with Aiden. Jack wanted Paul to be happy as much as Aiden did. Paul was the nice, happy sort of guy everyone liked. Not a big tough guy like Jack or the geek engineer like Aiden.

"Ready to face the Dragons, Paul?" Aiden asked. "That kicker of theirs is seriously hot!"

"The Griffins will kick their asses!" Paul deflected.

The team cheered from the showers. Jack lingered, undressing slowly.

"Paul needs to go bend over for that kicker. I swear he gets a hard-on every time Paul even takes off his helmet." Jack chuckled.

Aiden felt better, except he kept stealing glances at Jack's body while he stripped. They'd seen each other in the shower and changing in the locker rooms. Why did he need to stare every time? He'd seen dozens of men naked in locker rooms. Plenty of men had been in his bed, but Jack made Aiden's body go on full alert. Maybe that was why they played so well together?

"Chemistry," he blurted. Aiden recovered quickly. "Paul, you and that guy have it. Screw the enemy and get it out of your system at least."

Paul wasn't the type for hook-ups, but it was the best Aiden had. The chemistry Aiden felt with Jack blocked out any other man for him. They'd played on the Griffins' team for a few years, but Aiden had been spotty until he'd moved up in his company. Working less overtime meant he could devote more time to practice and games. Finally he'd earned the spot of starting quarterback and nothing was going to stop him.

"I'm not into random sex or I'd take you two home and teach you a lesson." Paul hopped into the shower section.

"Oh, the teacher is getting nasty," someone called from the showers.

Aiden laughed and locked eyes with Jack, but he wasn't smiling.

"You don't need me crashing the party," Jack shouted so Paul could hear him.

The idiot! He couldn't really believe there was anything between Aiden and Paul? That was insane! Paul wanted Mr Right and was no player. Aiden wasn't either. They had a brotherly vibe, just like Paul had with Jack. Paul was the one guy Aiden trusted not to grab Jack. Aiden had always wanted to be one of the popular guys and now he'd fallen for one. Jack had a new boyfriend all the time and left Aiden jealous.

"I'm not interested in doing either one of you. Clearly you need a tutoring session in grabbing what's in front of you. If you need a referee your first round, I'll volunteer. But I don't get in between the real deal," Paul said.

Whistles and hoots came from the showers. Not all of the men were gay, but they were a team. They made the team because of their skills, but worked together and bonded for the love of the game. Aiden didn't like his personal life, or lack thereof, being the butt of jokes in the locker room, but Jack was the only one who could fix it.

Men began to filter out, dressing quickly and nodding. Aiden got out a roll of tape for his ribs after his shower. He needed to be stronger so Jack would see he wasn't some geek in a cushy office. Jack's job screamed manly. A UPS driver had to lift boxes and navigate in crazy traffic. That uniform, just like the Griffins' silver and purple, turned Aiden on when Jack was in it.

Paul exited the shower and dried off quickly. "Maybe if you two let your own damn chemistry out of your dirty jock straps and go for it we'd all be happier? We'd all have less bitching and more fun. I'd rather watch you two make out than take cheap shots at each other. We need our quarterback and wide receiver working together."

"It all works out on the field," Aiden pointed out.

"If things change, it might blow up and make things worse," Jack returned. "We're all on the same team. You can go for the kicker and if it goes wrong, no harm done because they're still our rivals."

"We'll work it out. Jack's right about the other guy, Paul. We're on your side even if you fall for a Dragon." Aiden's ribs had ceased throbbing so he bent over and took off everything from the waist down.

"You two okay in here?" Paul asked.

Aiden looked around. The locker room had cleared out. He and Jack still needed to shower. Aiden's cock throbbed, but he kept a towel in front of himself. "Fine."

"We're adults. It's just teammate crap. Can't take the hits, stay off the field. He knows I don't mean it." Jack patted Aiden's shoulder.

"Sure." The touch made Aiden's body tingle. Aiden hated the rollercoaster. He needed more than teasing and touchdowns from Jack. They only communicated clearly in uniform.

"Have a good one, guys." Paul left the locker room.

Putting his gear away, Aiden headed for the shower. As he passed, Jack bent over to pick something up. Ignoring Jack's naked and very tight ass, Aiden kept walking. He'd been rejected by plenty of hot macho men who thought a muscled geek was still nothing but a geek. He wasn't about to make a fool of himself and lose a whole team of friends because of his deep attraction to Jack.

* * * *

Jack watched Aiden walk into the shower. That strong body had taken a lot of hits. As Aiden washed his black wavy hair, those blue eyes were closed and Jack could look all he wanted. Teasing was how he dealt with the attraction. He wasn't exactly from a family or background that talked about feelings.

When Aiden was rinsing the soap from his hair, he turned just enough to give Jack a glimpse of his stiff dick. It had to be Paul turning Aiden on. Telling himself lies was the way Jack survived and helped him avoid some pain at least. If Aiden and Paul hooked up, Jack would know Aiden had a good guy and could deal with it. Joking about the kicker in the Dragons defused the pressure.

Walking into the showers, Jack left only one spot between them despite a wide bank of free shower heads. The view made him hard as Aiden lathered his chest and the spray sent the suds south through his chest hair and around his erection. Jack washed his hair quickly and rinsed, hoping Aiden would be staring at him. Damn, that smart guy in a hot body kept his eyes down. It wasn't fair to give a guy everything. Good looks and a big brain. Fine, so Aiden wasn't a male model, but his face was far from ugly.

And his body! That athletic form deserved to be admired. Jack stared at the bruise and wanted to beat the crap out of whatever Dragon had given that to Aiden. He'd been taught better sportsmanship than that so he'd never take a cheap shot. Still he really wanted to kiss that bruise, not bust Aiden's balls about the pain.

"How are the ribs?" Jack asked.

Aiden looked over and shrugged. "Don't bother. I'll be fine." When he reached to try and wash his back, even with the hand opposite his bruise, the muscles pulled and Aiden cursed.

"Let me." Jack turned off his water, grabbed Jack's washcloth, and soaped it good before Aiden could even object.

"I can manage." Aiden's mouth said no, but his body relaxed under Jack's touch.

Jack grinned and took his time on Aiden's powerful shoulders. He had decent force, but his accuracy at throwing had earned him the starter spot. Jack wanted to kiss Aiden's neck but moved lower to scrub the sweat off his back.

"Sure, pull a muscle and you'll blame me." Jack worked the small of Aiden's back and started at his round ass. The urge to take Aiden pounded in Jack. Aiden's cock was as hard as Jack's. There was no denying it.

"I won't. Stop giving me crap and the Paul jokes. You know better." Aiden planted his hands on the wall of the shower and let the spray run over his face.

Washing Aiden's firm ass earned Jack a gasp from his sexy teammate. "What are you doing?"

"Stopping the jokes." Jack bit Aiden's shoulder and reached a hand around. Gripping the base of Aiden's cock, Jack had to look at the prize to truly enjoy him. "Don't fight it."

"Don't toy with me." Aiden turned and pushed Jack to arm's length as he leaned on the shower wall.

"Are you hard for Paul? Or for me?" Jack demanded as he turned off the water.

"Shut up with that! You know he's just a friend. If you're doing this to one-up Paul, stop. I'm not interested in sex games." Aiden's hands squeezed Jack's chest.

Jack smiled — at least Aiden was touching him. The man was a good liar! Truly he was cut out for corporate life. Aiden's hands were over Jack's nipples and the stimulation went straight to his cock.

"I believe you're just friends with Paul. I believe you don't want sex games. But I don't believe you want me to stop."

"What is wrong with you?" Aiden asked.

There was only one answer and Jack couldn't say it. Instead he tried to lean in and kiss Aiden. Damn the muscled arms of a quarterback! Denied genuine affection, Jack went the other way. He knelt and sucked Aiden's balls into his mouth before Aiden could react with more than a moan.

When Aiden's hips lifted, Jack licked up Aiden's thick member and teased the tip. The torment continued until Aiden grabbed Jack's head and guided his mouth down onto the shaft. Aiden gasped when Jack took it all, but neither of them were exactly new at this. Jack loved the rush of being nervous. If it weren't Aiden, it wouldn't matter.

"You bastard!" Aiden looked down at Jack.

Jack released Aiden's cock and stared up at him while nuzzling Aiden's sac. "You don't want it?"

"Shut up!" Aiden held Jack's head and rubbed his cock all over Jack's face. Kissing and licking the erection, Jack loved the feel of that man's cock pulsing for him.

"You think about me at night? On the field? You know you want it!" Jack nipped at the shaft as Aiden struggled with his lust.

"You just said it could ruin everything." Aiden shook his head.

"You never listen to me. Tell the truth for a change. Say you want me to fuck your brains out and take you home. You want me to suck your cock and then pound your ass." Jack loved seeing Aiden dirty. A muddy game gave him the best fantasies. But really he wanted to see Aiden let that guard down and be real. The guy never let his soft spot show, except on his body.

Jack gently touched around the bruise then slid his hands up Aiden's chest and pinched his nipples.

"Shut up." Aiden filled Jack's mouth with cock again.

To Jack's surprise and arousal, Aiden fucked his mouth like it was a glory hole. Jack could take anything the geek dished out and tongued that cock while Aiden took what he wanted. His face scrunched in determination, Aiden held Jack's head. Jack never broke eye contact, staring at his quarterback so Aiden wouldn't go into denial.

One of Jack's hands stayed up on Aiden's chest, pinching his nipple and tugging on chest hair to spur Aiden on. But Jack let his other hand slide down and cup Aiden's balls, rolling and tugging them. He wanted to know every inch of Aiden's body not just by sight but by feel. Where was he tender, ticklish and turned on? This was a good start. Jack rubbed behind Aiden's sac and the groaning grew serious.

Jack backed off to suck the tip and Aiden didn't fight it. The guy was too close. "Come for me," Jack urged.

There was no avoiding it now for Aiden. Seconds later, cum coated Jack's tongue and he got a rush of triumph. Aiden shuddered and his cock slid out, giving Jack another shot of cream to the chest.

"Shit! Jack." Aiden rested his head on the gleaming white tile.

Swallowing the prize, Jack stood up and grabbed Aiden's head for a change. Pulling him in, Jack took the kiss he'd been denied. Aiden didn't fight this time, wrapping his arms around Jack's torso.

Jack forced himself not to hold Aiden too tight. Aiden's ribs were still hurt and while some rough play in sex was fun, he didn't want to send the wrong message to Aiden. Chest to chest, Jack rubbed to feel the friction of the hair. Most of the men he'd dated were hairless guys. Jack needed a real man. Their tongues duelled for control, but Jack held Aiden's head and slowed the kiss to bring them back down to earth.

"I'm not hurting your ribs, am I?" Jack asked.

Aiden looked away. "I'm fine."

"I'm sorry. You really should give them a rest." Jack kissed Aiden's cheek.

"I had an X-ray. They're not broken." Aiden reached down and gripped Jack's hard cock. "What the hell are we doing?"

"Paul's always given us good advice before. If we turn each other on so much and get along, what the hell are we doing avoiding it?" Jack shrugged.

"If it's a joke, I'll quit and join the Dragons." Aiden's lips twitched.

"You wouldn't. The team would kill me. We're never going to be best friends because of this. So why fight it?" Jack kissed Aiden's neck.

"This shouldn't go to waste." Aiden stroked Jack's cock.

"Don't waste it. Stop playing and take it." Jack slapped Aiden's hand away. "I said I'm going to fuck you and I meant it. I'll never survive on just a blow job now. Come on. I'll make you come again."

Aiden pushed away from the wall and held onto Jack's shoulders. "You better." Aiden kissed Jack and the rush of triumph was like three touchdowns in one game.

Leading Aiden out of the showers, Jack grabbed a towel and wondered why he'd waited so long. Maybe his geeky teammate wasn't as stuffy and confident as Jack had built in his head. Seeing where Aiden worked daily had left an impression on Jack. Luckily they were naked now, and nothing mattered but the reality that they needed each other.

Chapter Two

Aiden damn near pinched himself as he dried off Jack. The sometimes-jerk had always been a good teammate and fair. What had pushed them from teasing to this? Aiden couldn't figure out. Was it just lust Jack needed to burn off?

When Jack sucked on Aiden's nipples, he couldn't care about anything else. Jack bit too and Aiden pressed in, knowing he'd give in to whatever Jack had planned. Jack loved to put Aiden in the Ivy League box, but a good education didn't mean he didn't like it rough and dirty as well.

Squeezing Jack's sac, Aiden moved in so he could kiss him. That made it real. The way Jack kissed was more intense than he'd imagined and Aiden had imagined it plenty!

"Are you going to fuck me or play with me all night? The cleaning crew will come in here eventually." Aiden didn't want to be discovered by the college kids this locker room really belonged to or a nice bunch of cleaning women who worked hard enough without being delayed by horny men humping.

"Ready?" Jack's hands spread Aiden's ass with confidence.

Jack fingered Aiden's ass until he groaned. Stealing another slow kiss, Aiden relaxed. He loved a confident man in bed. Too many college hook-ups that he'd hoped would grow had ended as one-night stands, yet Aiden's romantic side refused to give up.

Tired of getting hurt over and over, he'd thrown himself into football to take up his time but here he was again. Aiden broke the kiss and prayed Jack had protection in that locker of his. Jack nudged Aiden down on the bench and grabbed two packets from his locker.

When Aiden started to go face down, Jack grabbed him. "No way. On your back. I'm not straining your ribs one bit."

"I'm fine." Aiden's cock grew hard at the idea of fucking and watching it. Most men loved to do him doggie-style fast and the sex was over.

"I like watching you come." Jack pushed Aiden until his back was flat on the wooden bench. "Don't fight me. Unless you really like it rough."

Aiden smiled. "You think I don't?"

Jack tucked a few clean towels under the small of Aiden' back and gave his cock a quick lick. Then Aiden watched Jack slide on the protection and rip open another packet.

"I don't need much lube. What am I, a teenager?" Aiden mocked.

"It makes it better." Jack coated Aiden's hole with the slippery gel.

"Do it, quit teasing me!" Aiden gripped the wooden bench and tried to pretend his dick wasn't rock hard again already.

"You like me a lot." Jack kissed Aiden's sac. "Wait until we're done."

"Big talk. Prove it." Aiden smirked at Jack.

Then it finally started. Two big thumbs worked on his hole. Aiden flexed those muscles to show just how eager he was. Jack pressed his cock into Aiden and that long member slowly stretched his ass. Aiden closed his eyes for a second as his body adjusted. Then he forced himself to look to be sure. It was Jack inside him, inflicting short, hard thrusts then proceeding slowly deeper.

"Damn tease!" Aiden grumbled as his hips rocked for more.

"Not for long." Jack filled Aiden all the way and grabbed his erection.

The double impact made his hips lift as Jack possessed his body. Jack knelt on the bench instead of standing and Aiden gasped at the angle change. He took more of that already long shaft stretching his ass.

"You've been waiting for this. Waiting for me?" Jack rocked into Aiden's ass, steady but hard.

Aiden gasped at the building pressure and held onto the bench. "Yes, damn it!"

Pinching Aiden's nipple, Jack ground into his ass. Aiden's back arched as pleasure shot in every direction.

One of Jack's hands held Aiden's ass while the other pushed his shoulders back down. Aiden couldn't even feel if his ribs ached with so much sexual energy flooding his body. "Don't stop!"

Jack chuckled. "Your ass is mine. I never have to stop."

"Take it. Make me come, big talker." Aiden grinned as Jack hunched forward.

The man was flexible! Aiden watched intently as Jack's spine curled as he fucked Aiden. Aiden jerked his cock to torment Jack.

"You want it!" Aiden rubbed his balls.

"I take what I want." He squeezed Aiden's ass and leant forward even more.

The sight of Jack fucking and sucking him at the same time made Aiden's body tighten on the cock inside him. He couldn't take his eyes off the limber jock as his head bobbed down again and again, inflicting new pleasure on Aiden. Fucked and blown at the same time, Aiden couldn't believe it! Jack straightened up with a smug smile on his face.

Then Jack's hips went into overdrive. Aiden's insides ignited in spasms as Jack drove him hard. When Jack went down on Aiden's cock again, he shouted and tried to hold back. The pressure went from his ass to the base of his cock and back again until something had to give. Aiden shoved Jack's head off and jerked the tip once.

That was all it took.

Aiden's cum shot up to his shoulder. Then Jack took control back and sucked Aiden's member, swallowing the second round pumped from those tight balls. Aiden grunted and braced himself on Jack's cock because somehow the man never stopped fucking! Spent and sated by his own releases, Aiden watched Jack lean in and lick up the cum as those hips rocked faster.

"Damn it, come inside of me!" Aiden demanded.

"No!" Jack pulled free and tossed the protection aside.

Aiden grabbed the long erection and rubbed just under the head. Jack's body shook as he squeezed his own balls. "Aiden! Shit!"

The cum hit his stomach and Aiden ran his fingers through it. Stuffing the messy fingers in his mouth, Aiden sampled the tangy juice of the man he'd wanted for so long it'd become the impossible dream. Apparently it was very possible and they were actually compatible — sexually.

Jack had jerked Aiden's cock roughly even when it was spent and Aiden returned the favour. Growing confident, Aiden sat up and sucked the cum from Jack's cock.

"You call that rough?" Aiden rubbed Jack's cum into his chest.

"I didn't want to hurt your ribs. You want it doggie? I'll take you home and stack you on a pile of pillows while I abuse your ass for hours." Jack kissed him.

Aiden had to admit to himself that without the bit of lube, his ass might be raw right now. Jack's endurance was impressive. But that didn't mean Aiden would say no to another round. "I want to suck you off too."

"You will, but you'll be walking funny tomorrow. All those uptight guys in your office will know what you were doing." Jack slid a finger into Aiden's ass.

His tender flesh was reminded of how big and thick Jack's member was. Still Jack's words were more shocking. "I'm out at work. Who cares what they think? Fair warning, if you can fuck me that intensely, you'll never get rid of me."

"You think I want to get rid of you?" Jack pulled Aiden into a rough kiss.

Aiden let the other man take the lead as Jack nipped and licked his lips. Their tongues played, but Jack always won. Aiden's insides trembled with desire and intimacy. It might actually be real. Maybe he hadn't fallen for a jerk this time? Jack was tough on the outside, but Aiden needed to explore the whole man.

The kiss ended abruptly and Jack stared at Aiden. "You're not backing out?"

"What do you mean?" Aiden realised he'd tensed up.

"Coming home with me. Pizza and beer. We can watch a game on TV and see how long we can keep our clothes on." Jack bit and flicked Aiden's nipples.

Moaning, Aiden shook his head. "I'm not backing out. Any guy who can suck and fuck me at the same time must have more tricks up his sleeve."

"Good, now get dressed. Let's get out of here." Jack grabbed Aiden's hands and helped him up.

Maybe those damn ribs were the best thing that had happened to him in years? Jack actually seemed to care. Aiden couldn't wait to see Jack's place and be able to take all the time in the world to explore each other.

* * * *

Grabbing a pie on the way, Jack hoped his place wasn't a total mess. He lacked the neat freak gene. His apartment wasn't huge, or in the best building, but the sex had been so good that Jack hoped Aiden wouldn't care.

Jack opened the door and let Aiden go first.

"Cute." Aiden set the pizza on the basic wooden coffee table as Jack locked the door behind him.

"It's home. I've got beer or soda." Jack's confidence in bed and on the field was unquestioned, but he'd always been a lower-middle-class kid who tried to pass for middle class.

"How about a tour?" Aiden asked.

Jack nodded. "Living room, kitchen. The dining room is small, but I'm not big on entertaining."

There was a theme. The kitchen table and chairs were a butcher block-style wood that looked very durable. The couches were overstuffed and dominated the room. Aiden walked down the hall past the bathroom and to the bedroom. Following, Jack smiled at Aiden's easy-going attitude. The guy was too nice. The old bedroom set was refinished cherry wood and could hold them both. "One bedroom," Jack said.

"That's all you need. It's great." Aiden went in and looked around. He stopped at the banner celebrating the university they used for their football league. "Did you go there?"

Jack waited to hear that Aiden didn't think Jack had gone to college. When Aiden didn't comment further, Jack recovered. "I went a couple of years. It wasn't for me exactly."

"It's not everyone's brand of beer." Aiden smiled.

Lying wasn't Jack's style, but he didn't want sympathy. He changed the subject to something that was true. "I like what I do. I'm not stuck in an office all day. I stay in shape too."

"Great shape." Aiden leaned in and kissed Jack.

"We should eat before it gets cold." Jack grabbed Aiden by the hand and led him to the couch.

Heading back to the fridge, Jack grabbed a couple of beers, paper plates from on top of the appliance and napkins from the counter on the side. Setting it all on the coffee table, he found a game on one of his millions of channels. Aiden opened the pizza box and they settled down to refuelling after the workout.

"I should've taped your ribs up before we left." Jack grabbed another slice.

"I'm fine. Adrenaline rush." Aiden chewed on his crust.

Jack looked at Aiden's charcoal grey dress pants and crisp white shirt plus his glasses. He'd come straight from work, but Jack had seen Aiden like this all the time. In street clothes, like he wore before or after football games, he actually turned Jack on more.

"What?" Aiden wiped his mouth.

"Nothing. I just wondered. Do you really think Paul will get together with that Dragon?" Jack avoided the question he really wanted to ask by focusing on a mutual friend.

"I hope so. He doesn't seem to be dating anyone else. You never know if something will work until you're in it, but if he doesn't try, he'll never know." Aiden picked up another slice of pizza.

"Why didn't you hit on me then?" Jack sipped his beer.

Aiden smiled. "When I hit on men, I pick the wrong ones. Bad radar for good men. When I got my promotion and stopped the tons of overtime, I tried to date more. Ended up on an endless round of first dates. One-night stands. It was frustrating as hell. So I went harder into football and at least I can count on the team."

"And if we blow up it'll be weird." Jack nodded.

"Weird. But we're both adults. If we don't work out, we can still play. We're a good team on the field." Aiden set his plate down and took a long drink of his beer.

"We're pretty great in bed." Jack put his plate on the table.

"We haven't done anything in an actual bed yet." Aiden leaned over and kissed Jack softly.

Jack pulled him in and deepened the embrace. He loved how gentle Aiden could be. It was in how he threw a football just right and how he looked out for the new guys on the team. An engineer had to be exact and not put on too much pressure or things would collapse. As Jack coaxed Aiden close, he wrapped his arms around Aiden's muscles.

When Aiden's hands slid under his T-Shirt, Jack released Aiden and yanked off the shirt. He couldn't imagine anyone letting Aiden get away, but there were a lot of dumb men out there. Men who loved to date Jack until they found out he wasn't looking to move up in the company or give up the football league. Getting a boyfriend wasn't hard, finding one with a future seemed impossible.

Aiden kissed down Jack's chest while he worked on the buttons on Aiden's dress shirt. The feel of Aiden's teeth sliding over his ribs made Jack hard. "It feels like we should be talking more on a first date."

"We've been talking for a long time. Sex is what we've been putting off." Aiden ran his hand over Jack's fly.

Jack lifted and saw the genius of Aiden's logic. Grabbing Aiden's hand, Jack led him to the bedroom. "We'll talk later."

In the bedroom, Aiden opened Jack's fly and pushed his pants and briefs down quickly. Jack kicked off his shoes and reached for Aiden's clothes but was pushed back on the beige bedding. Aiden quickly removed his shirt, peeled off the undershirt and shoved his pants down. Stepping out of his shoes and the pool of clothing, Aiden knelt down between Jack's legs.

"No, get up here." Jack pulled on Aiden's shoulders.

"I will not be denied what I want." Aiden kissed Jack and pushed him back on the bed.

"Up here, at least where I can see you." Jack slid back on the bed.

Aiden climbed up but kept a hand on Jack's chest as he sucked Jack's cock all the way down. His body lifted, wanting to fuck Aiden's mouth, but after a few minutes, Jack surrendered. Aiden kissed over Jack's thighs, balls and stomach before going back to his cock. The deeper pulsing made Jack groan as Aiden eased his need.

Unwilling to give up for long, Jack reached for Aiden's hips and tried to pull him over. A stinging slap on Jack's thigh was Aiden's response.

"Come on, we can suck each other off. I swear, I'll fuck you still." Jack rubbed Aiden's erection with his hand and longed to suck on him.

"Most men love a blow job." Aiden pinched Jack's balls.

"Shit, I thought I was rough." Jack slapped Aiden's ass. Aiden's smile gave Jack so many ideas. "I could tie you up and fuck you all night."

"Go for it." Aiden slid his teeth along Jack's member and flicked the tip hard over and over with his tongue.

Jack lifted into Aiden's mouth and slapped his ass again. "If you weren't injured, I would. I'm not a sadist or a jerk."

"I know." Aiden kissed Jack's cock tenderly.

"Come on, you tease, get me off." Jack pinched Aiden's nipple hard and twisted. If nothing else, it made Aiden moan on Jack's dick.

Aiden backed off to suck only the tip and groaned on it. He rubbed the base of Jack's cock. Slapping Aiden's ass, Jack lifted up slightly to get more stimulation. The pressure snapped and he came hard, squeezing Aiden's ass. Jack screamed his lover's name.

Then Jack opened his eyes and saw Aiden's smile. Jack was going to return that favour and more. That teasing playful competition they had on the field worked so well here, he knew no other man could even compare to Aiden.

"Get what you wanted?" Jack asked.

"For starters." Aiden kissed Jack's member and licked his lips.

"Good. Hold on one second." Jack went to the bathroom and grabbed the tape he was so familiar with. He also grabbed some condoms and lube.

Returning, Jack found Aiden stretched out on the bed with a hard-on Jack had every intention of playing with. After he took care of his teammate, of course.

"Where have you been?" Aiden took off his glasses and set them on the nightstand.

Jack smiled and tossed the packets on the bed before kneeling next to Aiden. "Sit up."

"No, I'm fine. Don't stop the sex for first aid." Aiden kissed Jack's arms and neck as Jack pulled him up.

"You're too fucking strong for your own good. Don't fight me." Jack straddled Aiden's hips and carefully taped up the quarterback's ribs.

"I'm fine. You know, I think you want to ride my cock." Aiden kissed Jack's chest and pinched his ass to make it even more difficult.

"No, I like your ass." Jack added one more round than Aiden probably needed, but he didn't want to hurt those ribs. "Done."

"Finally. I'm going to lose it here. You smell so good." Aiden hugged Jack.

"Like locker room soap?" Jack chuckled.

"No, like a man. Maybe a little soap and pizza." Aiden pulled Jack in for a proper kiss.

Jack stroked Aiden's cock while he kissed the man. Before things sped out of hand, Jack turned Aiden over and settled him on a big pile of pillows under his chest. He kissed his way down that gorgeous back and inhaled Aiden's cologne. It wasn't strong, just a hint leftover from his clothes, but Jack had smelt it so often it turned him on instantly.

"Are you taking pictures back there?" Aiden teased.

Smacking Aiden's gorgeous ass felt good. Jack kissed the spot and slapped his flesh again. Men patted each other on the ass in football. It wasn't that kinky. But Aiden's big cock quickly stole Jack's attention. Opening the lube, he put just a drop in his palm and gripped Aiden's erection, jerking it slowly.

"Fuck! A hand job? You're a tease, Jack." Aiden moaned.

Hearing his name from Aiden's lips spurred Jack's efforts. A drop of lube on Aiden's pucker and Jack rubbed it in with his thumb. Aiden's body opened without hesitation. The trust here was so strong that Jack would bet he could tie Aiden up and fuck him senseless. That wasn't what Jack needed just then. He let go of Aiden's asshole and watched his body close.

Kissing Aiden's ass, he tongued over the opening and felt the muscles relax. Jack went lower, lapping Aiden's crack from bottom to top then back to that tempting hole. When his tongue pushed in, Jack felt Aiden push back.

Jack jerked on Aiden's cock fast and tongued his ass until he felt real tension in that horny geek. "Come for me. Come on." He slapped Aiden's ass and felt him flinch.

"Jack!" Aiden's hips snapped.

The cum slid over Jack's fingers as he tongued a circle around Aiden's asshole inside then outside of his body. Aiden shuddered and pushed back. "Damn it."

"Like the warm-up?" Jack pinched Aiden's ass.

"Hell yes. Please tell me you're hard." Aiden rolled onto his side and smiled up at Jack.

His cock strained for attention. "You think I could do that to you and not get it up?" He licked the cum off his hand and stretched out next to Aiden. "What do you want me to do with it?"

Aiden grinned and Jack swore the guy blushed. Jack kissed above the bruise where the tape was and dropped kisses up and up to Aiden's mouth.

Three hours later, Jack turned and woke up when Aiden wasn't pressed against him. Jack's body felt used in a good way and he hoped his new lover hadn't panicked and left. It had been a wonderfully sex-filled night.

Looking over at the nightstand, Jack saw Aiden's glasses. The relief made him fall back on the pillows.

Aiden walked quietly back in the room and Jack pulled back the covers. "No escaping."

"I didn't mean to wake you up." Aiden crawled back into bed and hugged Jack.

The change from the verbal jabs at practice to the affection now made Jack a little nervous. "I wanted you from the minute you joined the team."

Aiden rolled on top of Jack. "And you never asked me out because why?"

The real answer was complicated, but Jack wasn't sure it was the time to go into all the insecurities and details of a relationship so new. "You're not my usual type. Then we were so good together on the field, I didn't want to shake up the team adding sex into the equation."

"Sex can complicate things, but that's usually if it's bad. I think we're safe there." Aiden smiled. "We can't let it impact the team at all."

"You think they won't know?" Jack grabbed Aiden's ass.

Aiden shrugged. "They can know, but we can't let it hurt the game or team morale, no matter what happens."

"Don't get negative already. Paul will have a great time teasing us." Jack spread his guy's ass cheeks.

"Definitely. Maybe we'll inspire him to make a move on his crush?" Aiden kissed Jack softly. "I had a huge crush on you."

"Had?" Jack teased.

"We can take it deeper now, if you want." Aiden eased off Jack and rolled on his side, facing away.

"Of course I want it. I made the move on you today." Jack sensed the hesitation and cuddled in behind Aiden. Something or someone had bashed his confidence with men.

"About time." Aiden smiled.

Jack kissed Aiden's cheek. "I know. But you could've had me at any time."

"Sex isn't a relationship. If this isn't more, we shouldn't say anything to the team." Aiden pressed back to Jack. "Maybe it's too early to tell."

"Why don't we keep it quiet and see? There's a game on this weekend. Some friends from work are coming over to watch it. Want to join us?" Jack asked.

"I don't want to intrude on your group." Aiden shook his head.

Jack leaned over and bit Aiden's earlobe. "No, I want you there. You need to meet my friends outside of the football team. Do you have some other plans?"

"No." Aiden smiled. "Fine. I'll bring the beer."

"Good. I promise I won't screw you with the guys in the apartment." Jack kissed Aiden's neck.

"You'll wait until after the game and they go home?" Aiden chuckled.

"Definitely. Now go to sleep so we have time to fool around in the morning." Jack yawned.

"Tease," Aiden grumbled.

"I have to keep you wanting more," Jack said.

Chapter Three

Aiden parked in front of Jack's apartment building in the guest area. After work he'd stopped home to change his clothes and grab the case of beer. Meeting Jack's friends was a real relationship step and he didn't want to screw it up. They were different types, no doubt. Getting along on the field and in bed didn't always mean they'd fit into each other's lives.

Now it seemed obvious to Aiden why Jack had held off. The hope of something was better than seeing it not work. It was a bit defeatist, but Aiden had had enough rejection to sympathise. The Griffins meant a lot to Jack and Aiden. The connections would make it easier or harder.

Aiden headed up the stairs and knocked. Jack opened the door with a smile. Aiden handed over the beer and spotted three guys. Seeing Paul in the group was reassuring. The other two guys were from Jack's work, Will and Carl.

"So, Jack finally has a boyfriend he'll bring around us?" Carl asked.

Aiden grabbed a beer and a few slices of pizza from the kitchen. The three guests had the couch and all that was left was half of the loveseat with Jack or the recliner. Aiden chose the loveseat. "He's always talking about the guys he's dating at practice. You never meet them?"

Paul shrugged. "They weren't sure you existed. I seriously checked the calendar for April Fools when Jack said you two got involved."

"It's all your fault. You challenged him or something." Aiden grinned and started eating.

"Oh please, you were begging for it." Jack slid an arm on the back of the loveseat.

It felt real and Aiden liked it. Being so close to Jack was comfortable. The men ate and watched the game, shouting and cursing for their side. At half time they stretched and reloaded on beer and food.

"I still don't believe you two." Paul leaned on the kitchen counter.

"We'll see." Aiden shrugged, trying not to smile too big. "You should try it."

"No, I mean I don't believe it. I need to see some actual physical affection first. The body language is better, less hostile," Paul said.

"You really don't believe it?" Aiden chuckled. "Wow!"

"No making out while watching football. New rule," Carl announced.

Jack threw a pillow at him. "We can control ourselves. Paul's the one asking for it. While he spends half of every football game we play gawking at the kicker on the Dragons."

"Now we're a unified force. Look out." Aiden punched Paul's shoulder playfully.

"I've created a monster!" Paul grabbed another beer and went back to the couch with a bag of chips.

"You missed the pre-game, Aiden. We could've been torturing Paul longer." Jack patted the cushion on the loveseat.

Aiden sat willingly. "Sorry, I had to get the oil changed in my car. I kept putting it off."

"What kind of car?" Will asked.

"Lexus SUV." Aiden watched as eyebrows raised and eyes darted sideways. "It's only the RX."

Paul jumped in. "Anything made by Toyota lasts forever."

"Yeah." Carl nodded. "You don't change your own oil?"

Aiden held in a laugh. "No, I'm a nuclear engineer. Cars aren't my area."

"Nuclear? Like plants?" Will asked.

"Sure, but I actually work for the medical side of that. There are a lot of uses if we can handle it safely. But it's pretty boring conversation." Aiden realised there was a rather large gap if they were going to talk about work. "So what don't I know about Jack?"

Paul grinned. "I think you know him pretty well."

"He outranks us at UPS. He's been there forever so he gets those game days off and whatever," Carl said.

"Seniority has its benefits." Jack put his arms around Aiden again.

"Definitely, I couldn't really be on the football team all the time until I got promoted. All the overtime in the office and then the lab made it hard. Finally I can play." Aiden sort of half leaned on Jack, not wanting to get too cosy in front of two clearly straight men. He did like that Jack's group of friends was diverse.

"You're not radioactive or anything?" Will asked.

Aiden laughed. "No, they monitor the levels. There's an indicator on my badge. But we're dealing with really small amounts."

"So nice car, fancy lab job. You're really the quarterback?" Carl asked.

Aiden put a hand on Jack's knee when he tensed up. "I'm pretty good at hitting the target."

"Those two are linked in the head or something." Paul nodded. "We'd never win without them."

Will smiled. "Good. Jack needs someone who's good with his hands."

"He is," Jack said.

"I need some cheerleaders to come on screen," Carl teased.

"Anyone want soda for a change? I've had enough beer." Aiden headed for the kitchen.

"I'm good," Will replied.

"Me too!" Carl opened another beer.

"I'll have one." Paul looked back.

"I'll help him." Jack joined Aiden in the kitchen.

"I'm not tough enough to handle two sodas?" Aiden closed the fridge and turned.

"Paul wants a preview." Jack planted a serious kiss on Aiden who clutched the cans so they didn't fall.

The press of Jack's hard body made Aiden's tension melt away. It was real. He might not be a perfect fit, but no one was going to be a jerk. Aiden was trying and apparently Jack had noticed. Opening his mouth, Aiden let the kiss grow deeper only to torment Jack when Aiden slipped away.

"You'll pay for that," Jack said.

Aiden smiled at Paul. "Bossy on and off the field."

"He's like that at work too," Will said without taking his eyes off the screen.

"I don't need to know all the bedroom details." Carl waved his hand in the air.

"I didn't mean like that." Aiden handed Paul his can of soda.

Paul popped the top. "I'll have the dirty details later."

"He's just jealous because he's still going solo thinking of that hot kicker." Jack hugged Aiden as they stood behind the couch.

It felt comfortable. While Aiden had prepped some questions about UPS and their internal design to look interested and be able to talk design efficiency, he hadn't needed them. Those could help for a future lull when he knew the guys better.

"Thanks," Jack whispered in Aiden's ear.

"I'm glad you invited me," Aiden said.

"We are too. He talked about you enough." Carl shook his head. "Will and I thought maybe you might be some fantasy porn guy."

"I don't think I'm qualified for that sort of work but thanks. I think." Aiden frowned.

"That was a shot at me taking my time. And you definitely have what it takes." Jack squeezed Aiden.

Relishing the jolt of desire, Aiden predicted he'd be spending the night again and he was more than ready. Knowing it wasn't just sex but they could hang out made Aiden feel like they had real potential.

"You're thinking too much. You do that on the field sometimes too," Jack said.

"I'm thinking. In sports you can overthink, but now I'm good." Aiden kissed Jack's neck teasingly before going back to the loveseat.

Jack followed and pointed at Paul. "Look out. Aiden is plotting you and that kicker somehow. He doesn't have Ivy League degrees for nothing."

Sipping his soda, Paul focused on the TV.

"He's blushing," Aiden whispered. "He has to make the move himself."

Jack shrugged. "How much did he prod us? If you don't try, you'll never know."

Nodding, Aiden leaned on his boyfriend and crossed his fingers that their first practice as teammates and lovers would go this smoothly. Their spark on the field had followed them to the bedroom but hopefully the connection during the game hadn't fizzled from all of the sex!

* * * *

The next practice actually made Jack a little nervous. Would they have the same chemistry on the field? Aiden was supposed to take it easy on his ribs, but Jack had been privately keeping an eye on them. Taping up your own chest wasn't nearly as easy as someone else's.

Aiden was kept on the sidelines for most of the practice but towards the end of the practice session. "How about just a practice throw or two?"

Assistant coach Nelson shrugged. "If he feels up to it. We need to win the next game. Don't strain."

"I've been stretching a little." Aiden followed Jack onto the field and tagged out the second-string quarterback.

This time Jack wasn't at all jealous when Aiden squatted behind Paul. Jack knew where Aiden would be spending the night.

"You guys are so cute," Paul teased.

"Shut up and run the play," Jack returned.

Aiden winked at Jack and they got down to football. Jack was relieved when Aiden's throw landed right in his grip.

They were still good! Jack liked Aiden all the more after hanging out watching the game. He'd made an effort with Jack's friends and everything. The fear of Aiden being a secret snob was lifting, even if he drove a Lexus. Jack hadn't been to Aiden's townhouse yet, but he expected it to be equally nice.

He wasn't jealous or resentful. They were just so different and Aiden seemed oblivious to it. Jack hadn't brought the topic up either. The assistant coach called the practice to an end, but Jack tossed the ball to Aiden. A few passes later, Aiden was nice and loose. Jack ran over to him.

"Hurting?" Jack asked.

"No, I'm good. Having you tackle me with that rib tape daily did the trick." Aiden took off his helmet. "Can we get showered and go home now?"

"Sure. As long as you mean my place. I'm not done with your workout." Jack grabbed Aiden's ass.

Paul exited the locker room just as the duo were headed in. "Hey, everyone else is almost done in there, but maybe you planned it that way."

"Maybe." Aiden grinned. "Hey, Friday night I'm having a dinner at my place. Nothing major, a few friends. Want to come?"

"Sure. I'm late for something, but just text me what time." Paul nodded.

Jack almost got offended. "Do I get an invitation?"

"Sorry, I was going to bring it up tonight. I should've texted Paul tomorrow. You're the guest of honour." Aiden hugged him.

"So it's my turn to be in the hot seat?" Jack had to take as well as he gave, at least in the relationship arena.

"Yep. A couple friends from college and I get together once a month. Paul comes too sometimes. They're all gay so no worries about affection being weird. But they're a little geeky."

"I like geeks." Jack sat on the bench and undressed.

"Well, I'm the cool one of this bunch." Aiden smiled.

Jack wondered if he was up for that challenge. "The hottest, I'm sure, as well."

"You better think so." Aiden looked around. "This is weird."

"What? No one cares. We're not doing anything. And we're alone." Jack didn't want Aiden to freak out as things became real.

"I know. It's not weird that way. Being in here again. Where we first..." Aiden walked up to Jack naked except for the rib tape.

Tugging off the rib tape, Jack enjoyed the view. Aiden's five o'clock shadow had started coming in and Jack couldn't resist. Kissing his guy and feeling the scratch of the stubble got Jack hard.

"You can't wait until we get home?" Aiden asked.

Jack shook his head. "I want you all sweaty." Licking down the saltiness of Aiden's neck, Jack gripped his guy's cock and rubbed.

It took very little time for Aiden to get hard and thrust into Jack's palm. Aiden nipped and sucked on Jack's neck as Jack pushed his man against the lockers. Kissing his way down Aiden's body, Jack explored the rusty-coloured trail of hair down to his thick erection.

Sitting on the bench, Jack teased and moaned on Aiden's cock. Jack looked up at Aiden and saw the pleasure in his face. "You want me here and now too."

"I always want you!" Aiden's hips pushed into Jack's mouth.

Jack's hands slid around and pinched Aiden's ass, teasing the man Jack needed so much. "Turn around."

With a groan, Aiden faced the lockers and braced his hands on the metal doors. Jack ran his hands down Aiden's chest and guided his hips back and spread those strong legs. Naturally, Aiden tilted his hips to invite Jack.

"You're so sexy." Jack smacked Aiden's rear.

"Are you stalling?" Aiden asked.

"No, I want to get you good and ready." Jack grabbed protection from the locker and slid it on his own pulsing dick. Instead of diving in, he sat back and spread those round cheeks. Nipping and kissing the tender flesh, he twirled his tongue over Aiden's asshole.

"Damn, now! I'm not a virgin!" Aiden pushed back on Jack's tongue.

"I know." Jack worked both of his thumbs into Aiden's ass and spit in the hole. He loved to tease Aiden and that'd never end, he'd just change how he teased him. Jack worked more saliva on the opening then stood up. Pressing into his boyfriend, Jack wanted a little more friction this time. Aiden pushed back and moaned.

"Want real lube?" Jack offered.

Aiden shook his head. "I want you."

Jack wrapped his arms around Aiden's chest and filled his lover steadily until he could kiss Aiden. From their calves to lips they were pressed together as Jack's hips remained still, his cock buried in Aiden. Jack let his hands roam and pinch over Aiden's chest until he rocked back hard.

"Fuck me!" Aiden squeezed Jack's cock deep inside him.

"Impatient." Jack started with short thrusts. Then he gripped Aiden's cock and let it slide in and out of his hand as Aiden rocked back on Jack's cock.

"You like it?" Jack asked.

"God, yes! Don't go easy now that I'm your boyfriend." Aiden picked up the pace.

Jack let Aiden impale himself while Jack worked the throbbing shaft in his hand. Sucking the tip of Aiden's cock, Jack licked and bit Aiden's neck. Jack felt the tensing and how his lover fought for control.

"Give it up, come for me." Jack needed to hear Aiden's moans. He couldn't finish without Aiden's release.

"Jack!" Aiden panted and slammed a hand into the lockers.

The echo of vibrating metal mixed with Aiden's tightening body pushed Jack farther than he'd expected. Pulling all the way out, he filled that tight ass to the hilt twice more and tried to pull free as his release took over.

Aiden's hands swung back and held Jack's hips.

"What?" Jack demanded.

"You're coming inside me, I want to feel you." Aiden dug his fingers into Jack's flesh.

The intimacy was too much. Hugging Aiden tight, Jack moaned and grunted through the tight climax. "Aiden," he whispered.

"Like it?" Aiden turned his head and kissed Jack softly.

He couldn't lie. "Yeah. You don't want to be covered in cum?"

"When we're at your place and have all night to play, yes. I also like feeling you come inside of me. I think tonight I can have both." Aiden eased forward off Jack. "Quick shower and back to your place."

Jack followed Aiden to the showers. The sexy smart guy was a challenge and playful. Jack felt himself getting attached and falling hard.

He tried not to think about what to wear or talk about with the geeks. At least Paul would be there so Jack would have someone in his corner on top of Aiden. Rich smart guys weren't Jack's normal group, but maybe they wouldn't judge his old Honda or lack of college degrees if he made Aiden happy?

Chapter Four

The pasta was ready and Aiden pulled the garlic rolls out of the oven. Jack stood nearby dressed in black pants and a grey dress shirt, nervously mixing the salad. Aiden loved the sharper look but missed Jack's cute butt in jeans.

"You don't have anything to worry about. They're nice. Andy teaches at the University and Luke is on some government project he can't really talk about. Paul is nice and safe." Aiden took the salad from Jack and put it on the table.

"I know. You just didn't have to cook. Go to all the trouble." Jack sipped a beer as he paced.

"The guys and I sort of take turns hosting. It's not a big deal. Just my turn." Aiden checked the table then cornered Jack in the kitchen and kissed him. "It's pretty basic stuff."

"I'm not much of a cook." Jack shrugged.

The doorbell rang and Aiden opened the door. "Hi guys. Jack is already here."

Paul introduced Jack as Aiden opened the wine brought by Luke. Jack's tension disturbed Aiden a little, but he hoped Paul would calm things down. They weren't all in the same field. There was no reason for Jack to feel on display, though Aiden certainly sympathised. He'd felt a little scrutiny watching the game and he at least knew football.

Pouring the wine, Aiden watched the four men chat. Jack tried to look interested, but Aiden could tell he was bored. Aiden took the huge bowl of pasta to the table. "Food's ready."

The men came over and took their seats. They dug in and dished out the food. Aiden caught Jack's eye a few times. He didn't like the wine and kept to the water. Aiden wondered why his guy had left the beer in the kitchen but didn't want to make a fuss.

"So Jack, you're in delivery?" Luke asked.

"His friends were telling me he's got seniority," Aiden chimed in.

Jack shrugged. "I started right out of high school. Part time at first, during college, but then I liked the job. One time I needed to save up so I took a semester off and never went back."

"It happens. I've had several students leave. Tuition going up and in this a rough job market if you have a good income it's nothing to take for granted." Andy nodded.

"The job isn't exciting, but I get to play football on the weekends. Being stuck in an office or lab all the time wouldn't work for me anyway." Jack lifted his fork to his mouth and the pasta fell. "Damn!"

Aiden watched the piece of pasta bounce off Jack's firm chest and onto his plate. "It's no big deal. Let's put some stain remover on it."

Jack walked back into the kitchen. "Sorry."

"Stop it." Aiden grabbed Jack's hand and took him into the bedroom. "Here, put on one of mine and we'll let it soak."

"It's not a special shirt." Jack took it off and traded Aiden for a clean one.

"It'll clean up fine. So are you bored?" Aiden didn't want Jack to dread his friends.

"No, I'm sure they are. I don't know anything about museums." Jack shrugged as he buttoned the shirt.

"Museums? Like history or technology?" Aiden asked.

"Art. I know Paul's an art teacher, but he was talking about some guy who does stuff for the museum. Maybe he's showing his cultured side?" Jack checked the shirt in the mirror.

"You're doing great." Aiden hugged Jack from behind. "And I have no clue about art. Luke knows wine, not me. Everyone has their thing, but it's not culture or showing off. Andy's a drag queen on the weekends. You just need to get to know them."

Jack smiled. "I probably need to get out of my rut."

"Me too. But if Paul wants us to go to a museum, we're busy. I'd rather spend the day in bed. Let's get back out there." Aiden kissed Jack's cheek.

"Sounds good." Jack followed Aiden.

Aiden noticed the conversation die down as they returned. "What did we miss?"

"That shirt looks good on you!" Paul pointed to Jack.

"Thanks. Handy that we wear the same size." Jack went back to his dinner.

Luke cleared his throat. "We were talking about your email, Aiden. Complaining about the annual office party." Luke nodded to Jack.

"Office party?" Jack asked.

"They have one every year on the anniversary of when the research group was founded. It's a pain. Everyone brings dates and there's lots of drinking. There's usually a DJ. They rent out a big room at a fancy restaurant and it gets wild."

"Wild engineers?" Jack chuckled. "I'd love to see that."

"See, he wants to see it," Luke said.

Aiden's friends knew that he wanted a date for the party. He'd never had a boyfriend at the time of the party or it was too new or too near the end to take the guy. "I don't want to put him on the spot."

Shrugging, Jack looked a bit pale. "Let me know when it is and I'll see if I'm free."

Aiden smiled. "Sounds great."

* * * *

As soon as the guests were gone, Jack took off Aiden's shirt and set it on the couch. "I'm sorry, but I can't do the office party."

"What? I haven't even told you when it is." Aiden cleared the table and put the cork in the wine bottle.

Jack paced the living room and dragged his hands over his hair. "I don't think it's a good idea. That's moving too fast."

"Jack, it's not as if you can only bring spouses. It's not stuffy at all. It's open bar. Great steaks and a gift from the company. I just hate going alone every year." Aiden folded his arms.

Hating the hurt look on Aiden's face, Jack couldn't make it worse. Telling Aiden all the admins would know Jack because he delivered to that building might change Aiden's mind, but he didn't want to blow the whole relationship. They'd know what he did and see him in that uniform the next business day. Maybe if they'd been dating a year and established. Jack already loved Aiden and wasn't about to embarrass him.

"We've only been dating a week and a half. I just feel weird going so fast. Yeah, we've known each other for a long time, but we're going to tell people we've only been dating a week or two? That makes you look bad. Like you just brought a random date to have someone there and I might not impress them." Jack rubbed the back of his neck.

Aiden went back to the kitchen and worked on the dishes. The quiet scared Jack a bit.

"What? You're not going to talk to me now?" Jack asked.

"You made your decision. There's nothing for me to say, is there? I can't make you go. I'm not going to beg." Aiden loaded his dishwasher and added a soap packet.

"You don't have to make a big deal about it." Jack stood there stunned. "You're pissed?"

Aiden walked up to Jack. "Damn right I'm pissed! You made the first move. You started this relationship. Now it's going too fast? When it's *my* friends and *my* work, it's weird?"

"No, Andy and Luke are fine. We can go see Andy's drag show. I don't care, but the office thing is a lot of pressure." Jack had no idea how to fix what he'd done. Aiden wouldn't listen if he tried to explain the real issues and history now. Jack saw the stubborn glare in Aiden's eyes. It was the same look when he was out for a win.

"Pressure? Free food and booze at a nice party. All you have to do is make some boring small talk. I'm such an ass! Maybe you just wanted sex from me?"

Aiden went into the laundry room and returned with Jack's stained shirt and a Griffins T-shirt. "Here. You can give me the team shirt back at practice."

"You want me to leave?" Jack's jaw dropped. "I'm sorry, but I'm not ready to meet all your work people. Do you want to meet my mom tomorrow?" Jack couldn't believe Aiden had no fear about moving too fast.

Aiden folded his arms. "Family is a lot, I get that. But yes, I could meet your mom tomorrow and hopefully she'd like me. If we run into my sister at the mall, I'm not going to hide you. Now I think you want to hide me."

"No!" Jack pressed his fingers into his temples trying to stop the pain.

"Really? I think your football game probably has more guys at it usually. I think you trimmed down the guest list so it'd only be people who were okay with me being your boyfriend. Oh wait, maybe that word is moving too fast," Aiden said.

"Stop it. You're getting paranoid." Jack waved it off.

"No! I've known you too long to put up with your crap. You're hiding something. I don't know what it is, but I'm not playing games. If you just wanted a fuck buddy on the football team, you should've told me that up front." Aiden headed for the door.

"That's not it. We're different. Okay? From different worlds and there's no reason to rush it all." Jack didn't want to leave, but he knew Aiden wanted him out. He also couldn't argue that Aiden didn't know him well enough to tell he was holding back. But the truth was that with Aiden this mad, anything would get twisted and misunderstood.

"I've had a lot of guys reject me and dump me. I thought you were different." Aiden opened the door.

"I am. You just can't hear it right now." Jack stepped out onto the front step.

Aiden closed the door with a controlled anger. Jack had never seen Aiden this angry. Not even during their worst game, the worst ref call or the worst injury had Aiden lost his temper. Now Jack saw Aiden held all of his stuff in. How the hell would he fix this? Would Aiden even listen?

Chapter Five

Aiden went to the game very early and stretched in the locker room. The memories taunted him, but he hadn't taken a phone call from Jack in three days. He had called Paul to meet him here early. Someone had to make sense of this.

Footsteps echoed and Aiden turned to the door. Part of him wanted to see Jack, but he wasn't ready to talk sensibly yet. Paul appeared. "When I left your place, you two seemed fine."

"Thanks for coming early. I don't know what happened. That damn office party freaked him out." Aiden sat on the bench and let his shoulders slump. "He said it was moving too fast and all this crap. It wasn't even like I told him the date and he had something else."

"You guys are moving fast. There's still a lot to learn about each other. But I don't see the big deal about one party. He cleans up fine. Andy and Luke liked him." Paul folded his arms and pondered it.

"It's something else. He used the party as an excuse. You deal with kids every day. What's this passive-aggressive immaturity about?" Aiden asked.

Paul shrugged. "I haven't talked to him since the dinner. Have you?"

"No. I kicked him out and needed to cool off. Hell, I'm still mad. It's not like I asked him to move in or meet his family." Aiden refused to look at the shower where things had first changed for him and Jack. "I really got my hopes up."

"Maybe you shouldn't give up so quickly? Fights happen. You're such an engineer." Paul chuckled.

"Yes, I'm an engineer. What does that mean?" Aiden hated getting so worked up before a game, but he'd have plenty of energy to burn off.

"You're off or on. Something works or it doesn't. If it's not perfect, it's a failure." Paul smiled. "The rest of the world isn't black and white. People aren't perfect."

"I know." Aiden frowned. When things went south in a relationship he wrote it off. "I have friendships that have lasted decades. I accept people have flaws. He won't tell me the truth. We can't work through a problem if he's just going to avoid it."

"A fight is a fight. Try to talk to him now." Paul leaned on the lockers.

Aiden remembered leaning on those lockers naked with Jack. "I've always hung on too long. Hoped for more when it ended up a one-night stand."

"Did you tell him this?" Paul asked.

"No. He didn't ask. I don't understand how he met my friends, we're on the same football team, I can meet some of his friends—but he's not ready to meet the people I work with? Who cares? Aren't friends more important? These are co-workers. I just don't want to go alone. I told him all of this too. I was honest. For once I would have a date. A real guy I love."

"Love?" Paul whistled.

"Like. Whatever. If I'm out at work, I want to be able to flaunt a hot guy in front of the women there." Aiden hated sitting alone or dancing with the single women. Just like a family wedding, the pressure to be friendly and social only worked if you weren't lonely.

"Wait. Your office party would include all the admin and reception people there too, right?" Paul asked.

Aiden shrugged. "Of course. Who cares?"

Paul chuckled. "Ever see who delivers your UPS stuff at work?"

"No. Why?" Aiden's brain clicked the puzzle together. "You can't be serious?"

"It's on his route." Paul shrugged. "He's mentioned seeing you once or twice when dropping stuff off, but you were busy. I think that might be the issue."

"So the admins will know him as their UPS guy?" Aiden shook his head. "He'll sort of know them. Isn't that a good thing?"

"From your perspective, maybe. He never finished college. He drives a UPS truck and an old Honda. You drive a Lexus and make, just guessing here, more than double what he does." Paul sat next to Aiden. "Maybe he thinks he'd embarrass you. Or be a joke?"

"They're not like that. These are engineers and scientists, not Wall Street greed-mongers. Besides, he'd be there for me. I need someone. Whatever others think isn't the point." Aiden kicked the locker.

"I know men have been shitty to you. Jack's not like that. Not deep down. You know that and that's why you're upset." Paul put his hand on Aiden's back. "Talk to him. Show him you love him no matter what. No matter what anyone thinks about him. What he drives. Prove that he's not some delivery guy fantasy. He's not as tough as he acts."

"Neither am I." Aiden hung his head.

"You put up a good front. Successful, smart and athletic. We all get shot down and dumped. It's about the right guy, not every guy wanting you. Put all that high school and college stuff behind you," Paul said.

Aiden had confided more in Paul than he had in Jack, but that was the difference between a friend and a love interest. Sharing that with Jack could make Aiden look like a loser no one wanted. "I wish I was athletic as a kid. I had no coordination until college. Something clicked."

"Don't relive crap. Move forward. You're a great guy. Jack is lucky and so are you. I might be wrong about the issue. He might not be ready for a serious relationship, but I don't get that feeling from him. If he made the move on you, a teammate, he's serious." Paul hugged Aiden.

"Thanks, but there is always another option. He might've just been after sex." Aiden clapped his friend on the back and returned the hug, wishing it was Jack and things were good again.

The sound of footsteps broke up the hug and Aiden looked up. His stomach sank and any hope vanished.

A bunch of the teammates walked in, including Jack. He walked up and dropped the shirt Aiden had given him to wear home the night of the right. "Sorry to interrupt."

* * * *

Jack had survived being gay in school by being good at sports. No one had cared if he had a girlfriend or not if he made the plays. He had kept his love of men quiet until college then his life had sort of spun in different directions.

Avoiding Paul and Aiden in the locker room, he'd made it onto the field and in the game without dealing with what he'd walked in on.

The coaches were big on leaving personal crap off the field and working as a team. The head coach was out sick, but assistant coach Nelson took no crap. Jack watched as Aiden and Paul crouched. It was nothing for Jack to imagine them naked and doing stuff to each other. Jack hated that he'd fought with Aiden, but that man had a stubborn streak and hadn't taken any of Jack's calls either.

Taking off, Jack ran down the field and channelled his energy into the game. He didn't feel as connected to Aiden as before, but they could still win. Looking for the pass, he saw Aiden and their chemistry was alive and well. Jack reached out and picked the ball from the air. He hugged it to his chest and found a Dragon dead in front of him. Slamming into the guy, Jack held onto the ball as his body took the impact of the tackle.

The Dragon tried to wrench the ball from Jack's grip hard and the ref's whistle blew. The Dragon player stood and kicked Jack in the ribs. Jumping up, Jack ignored the pain and lunged for the other player, but the other Griffins held him back as the ref issued a big yardage penalty against the Dragons.

"Ignore him. You okay?" a linebacker asked.

Jack nodded. His ribs killed and he took a deep breath. The assistant coach took a timeout and Jack was on the bench with a paramedic, who worked every game, checking out his ribs. Jack looked for Aiden, but he was pacing the sideline like a caged animal. He went over to the linebacker who'd been near Jack and exchanged words.

"What's he doing?" Jack asked.

"Just rest. We'll let you sit out the rest of the quarter and make sure it's not more serious." The firm tone told Jack not to argue.

"It hurts when I breathe." Jack nodded.

"Sharp or ache?" the paramedic asked.

"Ache. I think it's just the muscles." Jack spotted Paul coming over.

"You okay?" Paul asked.

"Worry about your boyfriend. He wants to play more." Jack gestured to Aiden.

Paul shook his head. "You've got it all wrong. He's got you all wrong. You two need to talk more and screw less."

Assistant coach Nelson looked from Paul, to Jack and over to Aiden. "Off the field with that shit, guys. Play the game not your personal deals. Get out there."

The team hustled and Jack watched as he held the ice pack to his ribs. Watching Aiden and Paul so close again as they started the play hurt worse than any physical injury. He didn't believe Paul was really screwing Aiden, but even a friend comforting Aiden irked Jack. He wanted to be the one close to Aiden and hearing all of his secrets and fears. Paul was right, damn it! More talking and less sex. They knew each other, but there were deeper layers they hadn't hit yet.

The paramedic pushed water on Jack. "Is the pain getting worse? You look like you're in pain."

"Have anything for a broken heart?" Jack asked.

"No, but you'll probably survive it." The paramedic nodded to the team. "Tackle the guy and talk to him later."

Jack watched Aiden as he threw the pass to another man. The guy who'd kicked Jack tackled, but didn't abuse the receiver with the ball. It all seemed normal and the play was over. Then Aiden took off and rushed the guy. Jack stood up and watched in disbelief. It had to be a dream or a hallucination! But he hadn't hit his head. Aiden was avenging his attack?

"What the hell is he doing?" Nelson demanded.

Chapter Six

Mud splattered up as Aiden threw Jack's attacker to the ground and punched him in the chest. Aiden's knuckles throbbed, he rarely pounded men like this. Changing tactics, he went for the throat until the other Griffins pulled him off. The blind rage pounded inside Aiden. That Dragon asshole was going to pay for hurting Jack! The Dragon player rushed after Aiden, but his team held him back.

The ref blew the whistle, but the damage was done. Aiden was ejected from the game. It was an extreme move.

"They started this fighting!" Aiden shouted at the ref.

"Out. Now." The ref pointed.

Aiden went as his assistant coach rushed up and argued with the ref. Yanking off his helmet, Aiden heard his team and fans cheer him. Fights broke out, but that cheap shot at Jack had needed a better penalty than yards. Aiden walked past Jack without a word and went into the locker room.

He didn't feel better. Aiden wanted to get his rage out, but he loved Jack and was pissed at him. Punching the guy who had kicked his lover had felt good. Aiden had never fought back when he was bullied as a kid. It hadn't done any good now but it felt good. However, t didn't fix what was really wrong.

Slamming his fists into the lockers, he wanted to feel good again. One stupid party request caused all of his pain? Then he heard footsteps.

Jack walked in, stripped to the waist with an ice pack on his ribs.

"You okay?" Aiden asked.

"Nothing is broken. What the hell were you thinking going after the guy?" Jack sat on the bench.

"He kicked you. No reason, unprovoked. Asshole." Aiden yanked his jersey and pads off. The heat was getting to him.

"Yeah he is. So what? You deprived the team of your hands to prove a point?" Jack asked.

Aiden shook his head. "Throwing me out of the game was the dumb ref overreacting. I couldn't let it go. I had to stand up for you."

"I can stand up for myself. It's not worth creating a brawl over," Jack said.

"I was always the geek. Trust me, sometimes you need to fight back. Even if it's just to know you're not always a victim." Aiden peeled off the rest of his clothes.

"You're not a victim. You've got a great place, a great job and great hands. They're pissed because they're going to lose." Jack worked off his shoes. "You got bullied?"

"In grade school. I was a nerd. Too smart and not tough enough. It wasn't even about being gay." Aiden looked at Jack, so sexy and injured. "It's easier to protect others than yourself."

"Yeah, I get that. So you're not over me and onto a new guy already?" Jack asked.

"I think that'd be your typical move rather than mine. I'm used to getting dumped though. Plenty of times I get involved and it turns out it was just sex for the other guy. I'm not really what they're looking for, but I'm good in bed." Aiden opened his locker to have something to do.

"That's not what happened, Aiden." Jack leaned towards him and winced. "Damn it. Listen to me!"

Aiden turned. "Don't hurt yourself more. There's nothing to say."

"The hell there isn't! You still love me. You beat up a guy for me." Jack stood slowly. "It's not just sex. We've known each other so long that that was the missing piece, but that's not all it is."

"Then why? Why didn't you want to go to some stupid office party with me? I just didn't want to go alone. It's not an engagement party." Aiden inspected Jack's ribs to reassure himself Jack was fine. Paul's theory about Jack's work spun in the back of his mind, but he wanted to hear from Jack what was wrong.

"Why did you freak out over it? I say we're going a little fast and you're ready to pull the plug?" Jack turned it around.

"I think we just covered that. I got dumped. A lot. I lead with my heart and get hurt. Most of it was a mistake, I admit. My mistake. With you, though, it felt so real. Like it was more than sex and we had been teasing friends all along. Maybe the office party was sort of a test. Do you love me? Do you want me? Will you put up with this annoying stupid event that is a big deal where I work for me? Your answer said it all." Aiden rubbed his forehead.

"You read a lot into one event." Jack moved in closer to Aiden. "It's not moving too fast. I'd go to some family reunion or whatever. This is different. It's your work."

"So?" Aiden really couldn't believe it mattered what Jack did. "I don't care what your job is. They're not judging us like that."

"Aren't they?" Jack pressed Aiden into the lockers.

"No, even if they did, I don't care." Aiden wrapped his arms around Jack's neck. "I want you. It doesn't matter what you do. You're happy and an amazing person."

* * * *

Jack kissed Aiden because words just wouldn't do. Aiden tensed for a second before he gave in.

"I love you, damn it! That's why I'm so mad. This was different from those one-night stands and short-lived relationships. I don't want to lose this," Aiden said.

"You won't. I don't lose that easily. But you need to get it. I deliver to your building. I'm the guy bringing the deliveries. They'll know me." Jack had made peace with his job and liked it, but Aiden didn't need to have the admins making fun of him. Jack couldn't stand the idea of embarrassing Aiden. Who brought the UPS guy as their date?

"Good, you won't be as lonely if I get pulled into something." Aiden grinned. "You really think office talk would hurt me? Hurt us? I love my job, but what someone there says isn't going to change whether I play football on the weekends or date the hottest guy on the team. What could they say that'd bother me?"

Jack took a step back. "I didn't plan on it."

"Plan on what? Dating me?" Aiden's hands teased Jack's ribs.

Aiden's touch hit Jack in the heart. They belonged together. Jack rested his forehead on Aiden's shoulder. "No, I've been planning on getting close to you for a while. I didn't plan on this for my career. I started part time with UPS to help pay for college. I wasn't sure what I wanted to do, but my mom wanted me to get the college education and my grades were decent. Then my dad got sick a couple months into my sophomore year. Cancer."

"I'm sorry." Aiden held Jack tighter.

"Me too. He struggled for a year and couldn't work. Mom took care of him so she was off work too. I left college and went full time at UPS to help and handle the bills. They were great with the situation and my schedule." Jack hadn't talked about it for years. "I don't tell guys this."

Aiden kissed Jack's cheek. "You don't have to explain. But I'm not *those* other guys either."

"I know, I trust you. And you need to know." Jack nodded. "Dad died after about a year of fighting. Mom was a mess. I worked and took care of things until she needed to get back to work. She has friends and it keeps her occupied. Working gave me a routine and felt good. My mom tried to push me, but I couldn't go back to college. It makes no sense but because that's where I was when Dad got sick, I couldn't go back to that life."

"I understand. You had to grow up fast and take over. That student part of your life was over too soon, but life happens. I'd never look down on what you do." Aiden kissed his chin. "You've never complained about your job. A bad day sure, but you never sounded like you wanted to quit or do something else. If you wanted to go back to school I'd support it, but I've never heard you say anything like that."

Jack smiled. "I don't want something else. I just never dated a guy so close to my life and so different at the same time. It happened so fast. I was sure I'd screw it up."

"As long as we're together, we can't screw it up. Stay with me. Come to the party with me! Those admin girls will just be jealous of how hot my boyfriend is," Aiden said.

"Paul was right." Jack chuckled.

"You know nothing has ever or will ever happen with Paul. He's a friend. Like a brother. I was such a mess earlier that I asked him to come. I needed to talk it out." Aiden shrugged.

"Paul said we needed to talk more. He's right. We need to talk to each other not friends. Not yell or get mad. We can talk it out." Jack smiled.

"Maybe after we work out the physical needs." Aiden kissed Jack slowly and playfully. "We might need to wear ourselves out with sex first and then talk?"

The idea made Jack feel warm and oddly romantic. "You have a point. When we were fighting, I really wanted to kiss your mouth to keep you quiet for a bit. I'm not always good with words, but I know what I want. We can work it out if we just get the frustration out first."

Aiden kissed Jack's neck and let his tongue trail down his strong chest. "I can live with that. As long as we talk it out after the sex." He opened Jack's tight pants and pushed them lower before sucking Jack's cock all the way down.

Growing hard, Jack watched Aiden's every move. Those rough hands slid over Jack's ass and squeezed as Aiden tongued the underside of Jack's shaft.

"Not here. They'll come in."

"Let them." Aiden moved down to suck on Jack's balls. "Or you can come fast and work me over in the shower. We're done for this game."

"I could go back in." Jack arched his back as Aiden hit the sweet spot under the head of his cock. He flinched at the pain of stretching. "Damn."

"No more football for you today." Aiden's grip on Jack's ass tightened.

Jack gasped when Aiden swallowed Jack's cock all the way down and fucked him with his mouth. Thrusting in time with Aiden, Jack couldn't last long. He'd missed his guy so much Jack couldn't think of another man. Opening his eyes, he saw Aiden's and gave in to his lover. Pulling back, Jack came on Aiden's tongue and chin.

Grunting, Jack held Aiden's head. "You're going to be up all night. I'm going to fuck you senseless and maybe tomorrow we can really talk."

"We'll see if you can live up to that promise." Aiden sucked up all the cum before nuzzling his way back up Jack's body and pressing his hard cock to Jack's very satisfied one. "What are you going to do to me now?"

"Undress me all the way and let's hit the shower." Jack watched Aiden's erection bob as he moved to help free Jack from every stitch of clothing. "This rib shot does hurt."

"See, you were teasing me and now you'll have your turn." Aiden nudged Jack to the showers.

"You'll help me." Jack turned on the water and pushed Aiden under the spray.

"Get me off and I'll scrub you down." Aiden pressed his member to Jack's hip.

Jack grabbed Aiden's neck and kissed him hard. "I love you. No fight, no job and no teasing will ever stop that."

Aiden frowned. "I believe you. I love you too, even though you are really a pain in the ass. None of that other stuff even counts as an issue in our relationship, I don't care. Now get me off before halftime or we'll give the guys a show."

"I don't care if they see everything I want to do to you." Jack kissed Aiden and held him close.

"I don't want to torture Paul. He's got to get that Dragon, but we shouldn't flaunt our happiness and sex life. He's a friend." Aiden nipped Jack's lower lip.

Growling, Jack grabbed Aiden's cock in one hand and slid the other between Aiden's ass cheeks. "You're too nice. Maybe it'd spur him to make a move and get a sex life?"

Aiden moaned, but he couldn't reply. Jack jerked Aiden's cock, slipping two fingers into that sweet ass and pressing just right made Aiden's body press to Jack's. The debate was over for now as Jack fucked and stroked his man.

"Like it?" Jack asked. "You like being mine? I don't need to fuck or suck you to make you come for me."

"You're fucking me with your fingers," Aiden corrected.

"You like it better than my dick?" Jack pushed a third finger inside.

"No, hell, I don't know. I love you. Everything you do to me is great." Aiden held onto Jack as if he'd fall to the ground without the support.

Jack kissed Aiden's neck and squeezed the tip of his cock harder. "Good. I'll get all four fingers in you soon."

Groaning, Aiden shuddered when Jack tried to sneak his pinkie up there. "Sounds good, but not sure I can take that without lube."

"You want my fist, don't you?" Jack asked.

Aiden's eyes flew open. "I've never done that. I swear. I love toys, but your cock is massive enough."

"I like the idea of being your first fisting." Jack watched as Aiden's body kept on trembling.

Cum dotted Jack's stomach as Aiden grunted and moaned. "Jack!"

"I'm right here. You're not done yet." Jack pushed four fingers in and, with the orgasm, Aiden was open enough to take them. Over the third knuckle, Jack knew their fun was just beginning. "Your ass is mine. I've got toys too."

Aiden kissed Jack. "Harder," he said.

Jack went harder and deeper to hit the spot where Aiden couldn't help but climax again. The short groans and gasps mixed with how Aiden backed up for more convinced Jack they were a perfect match. More talking, but they could communicate and push each other physically. The trust was there and deeper if they only worked together.

"Jack!" Aiden's hips snapped then he went limp.

Kissing his lover's shoulder, Jack hugged him tight with his free arm. "I'll go to the office party if you really want me to. Just don't leave me alone with the wives and office admins for too long."

Jack slid his digits from Aiden's rear. Aiden hugged Jack tight. "Thank you! I won't let you go for a second. It means a lot to me."

The men kissed and Jack knew it was the right move even if going to the party still scared him a little. As long as Aiden was his, Jack could handle anything. "I'm not going to let anyone there grab my man. Now scrub me down so we can go cheer our team on."

"We're not going home?" Aiden frowned.

"No, we're going to sit on the sidelines cheering our team and go out afterward like always. Teamwork doesn't stop because you're horny and begging for a butt plug. You can wait until we get home." Jack kissed Aiden roughly as he washed Jack, being extra careful of his injured ribs.

"Fine, but I better not get any sleep until the sun comes up." Aiden squeezed Jack's fingers.

Carefully, Jack dislodged his digits from Aiden's ass. It felt natural to be connected, but in the old Irish pub where the team always celebrated, the most they'd get away with was holding hands. Jack planned on holding Aiden's hand a lot to remind himself that being together and fighting it out was far better than walking away and wondering.

"You don't get any sleep until after I've cooked you breakfast in bed." Jack smiled. "I can actually scramble eggs. That's about it."

"Sounds like heaven. Tomorrow is all ours." Aiden moved back to let the water rinse away the suds.

"Definitely. If we set a good example maybe Paul will get that Dragon as a boyfriend?" Jack found romance oddly hopeful for the first time in his life.

"I hope so. With us being all over each other, it'll grate on him being alone. Every time you had a boyfriend it made me nuts!" Aiden turned off the water.

Jack smiled and couldn't hide it. "None of them lasted because they weren't you. What an idiot, I didn't see what was in front of me."

"Yeah, we won't make that mistake again. I'd rather talk and fight than go a day without you again." Aiden led the way to the towels as the doors opened. The team piled in for the half-time meeting.

Chapter Seven

Aiden sat at the pub next to Jack as the team celebrated their victory. Somehow it felt even better that Aiden and Jack hadn't played the second half at all. The Griffins had won anyway while the couple everyone depended on had cheered from the bench.

"So you two are good? No more fighting?" the assistant coach asked.

"I'm sure we'll fight sometimes but not like that. We learned a lesson in this one." Aiden sipped his beer.

"Yeah, things will work smoother now." Jack smiled and nodded to Paul. "We just need to get him fixed up."

"Anyone. That Dragon keeps leering at Paul." Nelson chuckled. "What's his name? Rylan? Ryan? He's damn good at staring. Anyway, you're feeling better, Jack?"

"Well, we'll see how it goes." Aiden slid his hand over Jack's taped-up ribs. "The swelling seems to be better."

"Make sure to ice him up again when you get home." Nelson pointed at Aiden.

Jack shook his head. "I'm right here. I'm the one who taped up Aiden's ribs day after day. I can ice my own ribs."

"He'll make sure you do. Some guys are too tough and they need the push," said the assistant coach.

"Get used to it. You're in couplehood now." Paul chucked. "So cute I might puke."

"Shut up!" Aiden felt his cheeks go hot and changed the subject. He lifted his glass. "We're here to celebrate the win! To the Griffins, who didn't need Jack or I to slay the Dragons today!"

The team cheered and drank as their food arrived. Then things got quiet as the men refuelled. Aiden looked at Jack and smiled. Under the table, Aiden felt Jack's rough hand wrap around his and their fingers linked.

"Are you two thinking about moving in together?" Nelson asked.

Aiden wiped his mouth with a napkin. "We haven't talked about anything like that yet."

"Well, it is a money-saving move. You'd talk out your issues faster." Paul grinned.

"If you want to get all into the couple thing, get yourself a guy." Jack grinned. "Don't rush us."

"Exactly. When our leases are up, that's the logical time to discuss any changes." Aiden felt Jack squeeze his hand but not too hard. It was a playful squeeze.

"That doesn't mean we can't sleep at one place as much as we want," Jack said.

"Sure, once we try that out for a few months we can crunch the numbers on breaking a lease compared to riding it out. Plus where we want to live and how much room we'll need. There's a lot to consider." Aiden trailed his finger down Jack's palm.

"You got your eye on a guy, Paul." Nelson nodded.

"What if he is a Dragon?" Paul asked.

Nelson rolled his eyes. "There are bars full of gay men and you have to fall for a rival."

"I haven't fallen for anyone yet. Not really." Paul focused on his food.

Aiden could tell things were up in the air, but Paul was very interested in the kicker. Talking it over more now wouldn't do any good. Jack and Aiden had both eaten quickly. Stress and fighting burned as many calories as a game of football, it seemed. He finished his beer and pulled out his wallet. "We should go. Get more ice on those ribs."

"Fine. He just wants me in bed." Jack winked at Paul and reached for his wallet. "Ouch, can you get it, Aiden?"

"I got the bill. Take it easy." Aiden dropped enough cash to cover them both and their tip. "Come on."

"Pushy, rich boyfriend." Jack laughed as he stood up. "I'll get him for that later."

"You can buy next time. Save your ribs." Aiden didn't care about the money issue. Thankfully Jack was joking about it now. "You want to move in, that fuses our incomes and costs less. Who pays doesn't matter."

"Score, I got a sugar daddy that is young and hot." Jack kissed Aiden and the team cheered.

"See you guys at practice." Aiden waved and grabbed Jack's hand as they exited the pub.

* * * *

When they walked into Aiden's apartment, Jack kicked off his shoes and dropped his gear by the door. He pulled off his T-shirt and went to the big mirror on the foyer wall to survey the damage. "That'll be black and blue for a few days."

Aiden came back from the kitchen with an ice pack. "Yeah, but I'll baby you so it'll be good. I've set out a bottle of painkillers on the kitchen counter. They should help with the swelling too."

The cold made Jack shiver, but kissing Aiden fixed everything. "I'll be fine once I get you in bed. But for the record, I can pay my own way."

"Don't start a fight over a dinner. If we're serious about a relationship, then there is no mine or yours. It's all ours. I'm not going to get hung up on petty crap. No room for competition in a couple." Aiden hugged Jack tightly.

Jack smiled. "Good. I'm good with pooling things when we're ready for cohabitation and all that. But don't think you're going to treat me every time because you make more."

"Deal. Talking actually works." Aiden removed the tape from Jack's chest and inspected the bruise. "Are you sure you don't want to get an X-ray?"

"No, they pushed on the ribs good. If they were even hairline fractured, I'd have been screaming. It's only a bruise." Jack put the ice on it. "I might call off Monday. Lifting stuff will make it worse for a bit."

"Mental health day? We can stay in bed. Make it a long weekend." Aiden kissed him.

Jack laughed. "Mine is legit. Don't waste all your days to spoil me."

"I've got a lot of vacation time banked. I never use all my sick days. Maybe now that I've got someone to go places with a vacation will sound like real fun." Aiden locked the front door. "We've had dinner so maybe you need a nap? Rest those ribs?"

"You think you're going to get a rest?" Jack went to the kitchen and found the painkillers Aiden had left out on the counter. Shaking out four into his hand, Jack walked across the room, grabbed a bottle of water from the fridge and popped the pills.

Aiden slid up behind Jack and hugged him tight. "You wouldn't let me strain my ribs and now it's your turn to take it easy."

"Sex doesn't mean I have to strain those muscles. Get that cute ass of yours in bed. Naked. Now." Jack kissed Aiden briefly and closed the bottle of pills and the bottle of water.

Aiden strolled towards the hall as he took off his shirt. Then he turned and pushed his jeans down on his hips just a little. The teasing side of Aiden turned Jack on instantly. He followed his man down the hall.

Jack kicked off his jeans at the door and walked in with only briefs on. As directed, Aiden was naked on the bed. A bottle of lube and a packet of condoms sat on the nightstand. The fight really was over and they'd made peace with their love.

Sitting on the bed, Jack ran his hands up Aiden's legs and watched his erection pulse. "So when is this office party?"

"Next Friday after work. You can be a little late if you're working. I just want you to show up." Aiden pulled Jack on the bed fully and pushed him back on the stack of pillows.

"I'll be there on time." Jack watched Aiden tug down the briefs and toss them over the edge of the bed.

"Thanks." Aiden kissed his way up Jack's thighs, licking up Jack's cock and stomach.

Grabbing Aiden's hair, Jack pulled him up for a real kiss. Deep and rough, Jack held his man to him. Aiden moaned and straddled Jack's hips as his tongue worked in Jack's mouth. Their cocks rubbed together and Jack's hips lifted.

"I'm still going to fist your ass," Jack said.

"Tonight? You're a kinky freak." Aiden's hips rocked on Jack's body.

Jack held Aiden's face by the chin. "I won't hurt you. I'll go as far as you can take now, but I won't give up. The smile on your face when I suggested it was priceless. You're getting it."

"I think I should loosen up on something else first." Aiden slid a condom onto Jack's cock and lubed the shaft.

"I'm just your hunky sex toy now?" Jack leant back in the pillows.

"You're not straining those ribs." Aiden kissed Jack and sank on that big dick.

The tightness on Jack's cock made him lift as he slung his arms around Aiden's sexy neck. "You're doing all the work now." Jack stared in Aiden's eyes as the pressure and pleasure built inside them.

Aiden took the lead and rode Jack faster. There was no controlling Aiden until he had all of Jack's cock deep inside him. Jack let his hands roam over Aiden's athletic chest. The lines of muscles and sexy hair made Jack lift harder into his boyfriend's ass. The idea of the same man knowing every inch of him and what he loved made it so much better as Jack held Aiden's hips down.

Grinding on him, Aiden jerked his own cock. "I can't stop!"

Aiden came all over Jack's chest and he lifted hard too as Aiden's body squeezed in climax. Trying to hold out was useless for Jack as Aiden leaned in for a deep kiss. Intimacy and great sex? Jack held Aiden to him and thrust up as their tongues duelled.

Jack's release slammed his body hard as he muttered Aiden's name. "You're mine, Aiden."

"Damn right," Aiden said.

"You trust me?" Jack asked.

"Of course. But it's not a rush. We've got forever to fulfil each other's sexual fantasies and push each other's buttons." Aiden ran his fingers around Jack's bruise. "We could sixty-nine or just cuddle. No stress on your muscles."

"No stress on my ribs shoving a hand up your ass either." Jack nipped Aiden's chin. "If you're not ready, say so."

Aiden licked his lips. No man had ever offered that to him. He'd never had the balls to ask for it. "I want the whole hand this time up to your wrist. I've put plenty of good-size toys up there in my single days."

"Yeah, you can relax more than you do. Trust me." Jack tugged Aiden to lie across his lap.

Stretching out, Aiden turned his head so he could see Jack's face. Aiden tensed as Jack drizzled cool lube down his crack. He took a deep breath and relaxed his muscles so the lube slid inside of him. He had a good collection of butt plugs and toys. Jack wouldn't have to work too hard to get his fist up there.

Jack started with a couple of fingers and Aiden hummed as the digits woke up nerve endings in a new way. Fingers could tease inside the way a cock just couldn't and Jack knew what he was doing. He went from two fingers to four and deeper.

"God, yes!" Aiden pressed back.

"You've done this to yourself?" Jack asked.

"I've got toys. Plugs of all sizes. Not as big as your fist, but being single doesn't mean I can live without this." Aiden smiled.

"You don't have to worry about that now." Jack pulled his hand back.

The loss made Aiden sigh. "Prove it. Get me off like this."

"Don't rush it." Jack rubbed his thumb behind Aiden's sac.

Groaning, Aiden lifted and rocked back. "Give it to me."

Jack pushed in with a fist this time and Aiden gasped at the new shape. This was no toy that could be squeezed down, it was bone and muscle. Forcing himself to relax, Aiden welcomed the invasion. Letting Jack possess his body this way, the first man to do it, turned him on in a new way.

"Deep breath." Jack added some lube and twisted his fist slightly, then advanced another two inches.

"That's it. So good!" The stretching in his ass flooded Aiden's body with sweet electricity.

Jack turned his hand and eased back. "You've only taken half of it. Sure you want more?"

Aiden nodded and focused on relaxing each muscle as Jack pressed to it. Getting the pressure and the relief with the stretching and the heat made Aiden want more. This wasn't a toy! "Take me."

"Damn! What sort of toys are you stuffing up there?" Jack went farther this time and Aiden began to tremble.

"So good! I'll show you my toys later, but this is better. It's you!" Aiden arched his back and opened for more.

Jack pushed in and Aiden groaned. "Damn, I'm in."

"Like it? If it's not turning you on, you can stop." Aiden hoped Jack liked it, but not every guy got off shoving a hand up his boyfriend's ass.

"I love it." Jack twisted his hand and pulled back.

"Fuck me with it or it's not fisting," Aiden insisted.

He closed his eyes and took in the sensation. Jack's large hand worked in and out with confidence. A nervous guy could hurt him, but Aiden trusted his hunk. Jack changed from fist back to fingers first and Aiden shuddered.

"Good?" Jack asked.

"Fucking great! It's not your first time." Aiden didn't care how many men had enjoyed Jack before. He was Aiden's man now!

"It's not something I do every day." Jack spread Aiden's cheeks and added more lube before shoving his fingers and half his palm up there.

"Fuck me!" Aiden demanded.

Jack finally did, shoving that same part of his hand in and out of Aiden's ass fast.

The sweet stretching and pressure made Aiden's cock go hard. "Don't stop!" He bucked back on that hand as his release built.

"Come on. Come for me." Jack's fingers worked deep and hit the magic spot over and over.

"Jack!" Aiden came on Jack's legs as his insides quivered and rippled so deep he couldn't even believe it was real.

"Easy, don't break my fingers." Jack kept sliding his hand in and out until Aiden's body went limp, blood pounding in his head while the rest of him was spent.

Then Jack's fingers teased his crack. "Too rough?" he asked.

Aiden chuckled. "Perfect. You're amazing."

"I'm not the one who took a fist. That's trust."

"Love too. I came all over you." Aiden smiled.

Jack grabbed Aiden's hand and pulled it over. Jack's huge erection didn't shock Aiden. He was relieved Jack truly enjoyed the play. Aiden curled his fingers around Jack's cock and jerked off his boyfriend. "Like my ass?" Aiden teased.

"Love it! I do want to see your toy collection tomorrow." Jack smacked Aiden's ass.

"You can have the full tour of my house, every drawer, and you can tell me all of your fantasies." Aiden rubbed the tip of Jack's cock.

Jack shook and Aiden rolled onto his side to watch his man coming. The tough guy shook and grunted with no hint of shame. As Jack caught his breath, Aiden lapped up the cum. He kissed Jack and cuddled up to his guy. Kinky sex and sleepovers made it almost too good to be true! Luckily for Aiden, his ass would ache for a few days and remind him it was very real.

Chapter Eight

One month later…

Sitting at his desk working on boring reports, Aiden's mind kept drifting. His life was great even when doing his least favourite part of his day job. The Griffins were having a winning season and his boyfriend had moved in totally as of last weekend. Jack had proved pretty popular with the office staff at the holiday party as well.

His phone beeped and Aiden pushed the speaker button for the internal call. "Hi, Trish."

"Your *boyfriend* is here, Aiden," she said in a dreamy tone.

"Thanks, I'll be right out." Aiden got teased but in a good way. Jack was hot, masculine and strong.

Walking down the hall, he made the right turns to the receptionist desk. The maze of the office explained why he'd never noticed Jack was the UPS guy for their building. The women at the reception desk were drooling over Jack even more now that they knew he was Aiden's man.

"Hey, this has become my favourite part of the day." Jack kissed Aiden.

"I'm glad. Are you swamped or want to grab lunch?" Aiden asked.

"We're putting in a sandwich order now. Should be here in half an hour," Trish said.

"Great, turkey club." Aiden smiled.

"Today is pretty light. I'll take a roast beef sandwich." Jack shrugged.

"Sure thing. We'll bring it back." Trish waved at them.

"Thanks!" Aiden headed back.

Jack raised an eyebrow at Aiden as they walked to his office. "What's all that about?"

"The manager wants to ask a favour." Aiden rolled his eyes.

As if on cue, Mr Hendricks walked out of the hall where the big offices were. "Jack, always a pleasure." He shook Jack's hand hard.

"Thanks. I just stopped in to see Aiden." Jack slid his hands into his pockets.

"I know and you're always welcome around here. We're a family research group and I hope you can come to the office picnic this summer." Hendricks rubbed his hands together and grinned.

"Sure, I'd love to. Any special reason?" Jack asked.

Aiden smiled. "They always have a softball game against the group one floor down. He wants another ringer."

"That's not entirely true. We want to support Aiden and your relationship. Beating the other team with more strong athletes on our side is another plus." Hendricks nodded.

"I'm not much of a baseball player." Jack shrugged.

Aiden winked at him. "You can run, catch and intimidate them. Maybe if the group sponsored the Griffins that might convince you?"

"Then I'd have to play." Jack nodded.

"Why don't you put the paperwork for this sponsorship on my desk and I'll look it over. Come to the picnic." Hendricks pointed at Jack.

"Sure thing." Jack smiled.

Aiden steered Jack into the office and closed the door. "Sorry about that. But you can't say they don't like you. I've only benefited from dating the hot guy who drops by every day. The men wish they looked like you and the women wish their men did."

"I'm glad." Jack kissed him. "You really play softball once a year?"

"Not my favourite sport, but it includes everyone. The women weren't in for touch football." Aiden shrugged and claimed Jack's lips again. "I love you in your uniform."

Jack chuckled. "You're so weird. I look much better in the Griffin purple."

"You look best naked, but seeing you during the day, every day, is a wonderful break no matter how long." Aiden deepened the embrace with Jack. Some days Jack couldn't come back at all and was running behind schedule. Just seeing him was enough to brighten the day, but when he could stay for lunch, Aiden loved to prove just how gay-friendly his office was.

"We're not screwing around in here," Jack said against Aiden's mouth.

Aiden moaned. "You've got no problem doing things in the locker room but not here?"

"I want to remain welcome here. If you're working late and need a break that might be different." Jack nipped at Aiden's neck until he backed off.

Just then a tap on the door announced their lunch. Aiden grabbed the sandwiches and handed over the cash while Jack sat in a guest chair. After closing the door, Aiden set the lunch down and flopped in his desk chair unsatisfied. "You'll have to make it up to me tonight."

Jack unwrapped his sandwich and dug in. "I promise."

Aiden reached into the mini-fridge he'd put in his office and brought out sodas. "We'll see."

* * * *

Jack usually got home before Aiden and this time he made the most of it. He'd picked up a new toy and stripped down to nothing. Like clockwork, Aiden's key was in the lock at quarter to six and Jack slid the vibrating cock ring on but didn't give it any power yet.

The door opened and Aiden was talking to someone. On the phone? Jack looked and saw Paul outside. "Hang on!" He ran to the bedroom and yanked open a drawer to find some clothes. He heard Aiden calling as he came into the townhouse.

Aiden knocked on the bedroom door. "Okay in there?"

"Yeah, I forgot Paul was coming for dinner tonight. I'll be right out." Jack had got so into making up the office sex to Aiden that he'd forgotten the dinner plans.

Aiden opened the door. "Don't worry. Paul went home. Rain check."

Jack's shoulders slumped. "He didn't have to."

"You didn't have to run for cover either. He's seen you in the locker room. He figured that you had something special planned for me and dinner would just be awkward. What is this?" Aiden picked up the ring and the battery pack.

"Your surprise. If Paul's gone, get naked and I'll show you." Jack knew he'd be making dinner up to Paul soon, but right now he'd thrill his man. "I owe you for lunch. You wanted a nooner."

"That's sweet, but I'm going to get at least a blow job in my office before the picnic." Aiden stripped off his clothes and flopped on the bed.

"I don't want them thinking we're sex-crazed maniacs." Jack stretched out on the bed and slid the ring over his cock. Then he leaned over and tongued Aiden's member until it hardened.

"What does this do?" Aiden turned the dial on the battery pack.

The vibrations went from mild to unbearable and back. "Fuck!" He grabbed the pack from Aiden.

"Oops. A special new toy? Thank you." Aiden kissed Jack. "I think we'll both enjoy that."

"Damn right." Jack pushed Aiden up to the pillows. "Face down."

Aiden flipped over without protest. Jack took a second to admire his boyfriend's ass hiked up in the air while hugging pillows. Once he grabbed protection from the nightstand, Jack slid it on and leant down. Kissing and licking Aiden's asshole was just for fun. The guy could now take a fist or a wide butt plug without a second thought. Still Jack loved taking his time and working Aiden into a frenzy of need.

"Fuck me, you tease!" Aiden shouted.

Jack smacked Aiden's ass and spread those round cheeks. "I think tomorrow you should wear a butt plug until I get there for lunch."

Aiden laughed. "You won't suck me off, but you'll use sex toys on me? You're nuts."

"I'll suck you off before I take it out." Jack knew he'd never deny Aiden anything for long. Putting his own twist on it, he hoped, would turn Aiden on even more.

"I love you!" Aiden said.

"Me too." Jack thrust deep into Aiden's ass until they pressed the ring between them. It fit snugly and Jack turned the dial up a little.

"Shit, that's intense." Aiden ground his ass back on Jack.

"More?" Jack dialled up the vibrations a quarter turn and reached down to make sure it pressed right in behind Aiden's balls.

"Fuck me or I'll come in two seconds!" Aiden rocked his hips to vary the contact with the ring.

"You love it!" Jack pulled out and it wasn't enough. The vibrations without being inside Aiden made him nuts. Pounding Aiden's ass, Jack dropped the power pack and fucked his boyfriend. Jack leaned Aiden over, ground into the sexy man and kissed his back. Gripping Aiden's cock, Jack jerked his boyfriend off hard. "I need one of these on you."

"No, I can barely take this." Aiden moaned and trembled.

"I was going to get vibrating balls that go inside. I'll make you come over and over." Jack worked Aiden's cock faster. "You want them, don't you?"

At first Aiden shook his head, but as Jack kissed his neck and pumped deep inside him, Aiden nodded. "Please."

Jack's hips took over as he came inside Aiden. "I love you! Aiden, we don't need toys. Not right now. I just want you."

Aiden screamed into the pillow and panted as Jack felt his man's cum coat his fingers. That tight ass squeezed Jack's cock as they both gasped for air.

"I like the toys," Aiden admitted. "I love them when you're behind it."

Jack turned the toy off and slid from Aiden and rolled him over so they could kiss properly. "I like using toys on you too. This one was intense."

"We'll get used to it." Aiden ran his hands over Jack's shoulders and it was as good as the sex.

"You want more toys?" Jack kissed Aiden's chest.

"I want more with you. Whatever, whenever, wherever. Toys or none, with the right man it's always good." Aiden grinned.

"Fine, I swear if you wear that butt plug to work tomorrow, I'll blow you in your office at lunch. Okay?" Jack asked.

"Deal. Now about the next game." Aiden yawned. "I wonder if some sort of plug might improve my performance?"

"Run with one of those in? You think you can control yourself?" Jack felt the heat rushing to his cock at the very idea of it.

"Maybe. Maybe not, I'll be wearing a cup so there's some constriction there." Aiden bit Jack's lower lip.

"Let's see how you do tomorrow and maybe I'll encourage that experiment." Jack pinched Aiden's nipples until his man lifted. "I love you and with your dirty mind, we'll never get bored in bed."

Aiden rolled Jack onto his back. "I'll never get bored with you, ever. I love you and next time you go toy shopping, I want to go along."

"Fine, but I can buy presents for you on my own too."

"Definitely. I love this." Aiden pressed the ring to Jack's member, grabbed the power pack and dialled it up.

Jack's hips lifted off the bed. "Better than a touchdown?"

"Better than a million of those." Aiden chuckled and kissed his boyfriend.

Jack moaned as Aiden played with the dial. They were a hell of a team anywhere!

CROSSING THE LINE

Megan Slayer

Dedication

Flash — I'm glad you found the picture.
Cheryl — I'm glad you jumped on board with this.
Without you two, this wouldn't have worked.
S.B. — you rock and I'm glad you're my editor.
J.P.Z. — You make crossing the line so much fun, let's
do it again!

Chapter One

How come the right fit is never there when you want it?

Ryan Malone sighed and pressed the last glazing point into place. He wished he was working on one of his paintings rather than framing artwork for the local high school. The man in the painting stirred something deep within him, something exciting and unattainable. He tapped the point into the frame, double-checked the fit.

The man in the painting wasn't just any guy. No, Paul Toth surpassed most men. Gifted in the art classroom and smooth in social situations, he turned heads with his effortless style. Ryan flipped the painting over. Staring at Paul for the last two months had seared his visage into Ryan's memory. The guy had grace and damn was he cute. Brown eyes with just a hint of wonder. Thick, dark brown hair combed like he'd just walked out of a salon...and that body... Muscles where a man should be sculpted, but not boxy or bulky.

Thank God Ryan had closed his office door. Anyone passing by would've seen the bulge in his pants. On the outside, Paul embodied everything Ryan wanted in a man.

"But he plays for the other team," Ryan said to himself. His phone beeped, reminding him of his appointment with the principal. "I haven't met with a principal since I was in school." He chuckled. Thinking about school didn't make him feel much better.

He wrapped the artwork in butcher paper, then grabbed his keys. Thirty minutes later he stood outside Northwood High School. He pressed the button to lock his Jeep.

Just take the painting in, he probably won't be there. Ryan gripped the painting and strode into the foyer. Northwood happened to be the home of the soon-to-be-named Teacher of the Year, aka Paul Toth. He pushed the second door handle, but nothing happened.

"We need to buzz you in," came a voice over the loudspeaker.

Ryan cringed. He hated being caught off guard. "I'm Ryan Malone, here with the Teacher of the Year painting."

"Very good," the woman said. "Door's open."

Ryan headed to the office. The quicker he made his delivery, the sooner he'd be able to leave. Seeing Paul wouldn't help things.

"Mr Malone."

Ryan grinned at the principal. "Hello, Mr Laubenthal. I have the painting."

"Perfect." George Laubenthal rubbed his meaty hands together. His salt-and-pepper eyebrows bobbed and his moustache twitched. "It's been eating Toth alive not to be doing this for us this year."

"The painting?" He handed the principal the package. "I know he teaches art, but I wasn't sure if he created the portraits."

"Yes. Mr Toth has painted the last four winners. I couldn't exactly have him paint himself. Let's show the girls in the office." Laubenthal led the way to the main office. "Girls, you're going to love this."

"Well, we can only hope," Ryan muttered.

"Nan, see if the work room is empty. Don't want wandering eyes." Laubenthal placed the painting on the nearest desk. His eyes sparkled behind his thick glasses. "I'm excited to see it."

When the secretary came back grinning, George unveiled the painting. He picked at the tape holding the paper closed, then gasped. "This is fantastic." George stepped back from the painting and pulled an envelope from his coat pocket. He handed Ryan the envelope. "That's for you. Board approved. We truly appreciate it."

Ryan stared at the image of Paul and suppressed a sigh. In the bright light, the highlights in Paul's dark hair stood out. His brown eyes sparkled with poise and mischief. He'd folded his arms in the photo and Ryan had taken the opportunity to define his biceps a bit more. When he'd created the painting, he hadn't been able to tear his gaze from Paul's. Now, seeing the image with others around, Paul took his breath away. Paul embodied control and strength. Ryan forced himself to look away from the image that had haunted his dreams.

"I'm glad you're happy." Ryan nodded and placed the folded envelope in his back pocket. "I'd love to hang around and gawk at the painting, but I've got some other things to attend to so I'll be going. Thank you for asking me to do this for you."

"I'm glad Professor Pride suggested you." George Laubenthal offered his hand. "I've seen your work down at the NEU Galleries. We're honoured to have a piece here, as well. Thank you."

Ryan shook hands with the principal, then made his way out of the office. Only a few more steps and he'd be back outside in the safety of his Jeep and the seclusion of his office. The paintings never talked back and they sure as hell didn't go out of their way to break his heart. Paul, on the other hand, could do both.

"Malone? Is that you?"

Ryan stopped in his tracks. *Fuck in a monumental-sized basket.* He knew the voice all too well. Paul. Footsteps thumped on the tiled floor behind him.

"Ryan?"

Unless he outright ignored Paul, there was no escape. Ryan sighed and stopped at the door. "Toth."

Paul strolled up beside Ryan. "Thought I saw you here." A quirky smile played on Paul's lips, much like the one in the painting. "What's a guy like you doing in a place like this? I haven't set up any lectures for the senior art students, although since you are here, I should probably try to wrangle you into talking to them." His brown eyes glittered and the dimple in his cheek became more pronounced. Damn, the man was more handsome in person than any photograph.

Being so close to a man he lusted after wasn't safe for Ryan. But holy hell, being alone sucked ass even more. "I did some work for the principal."

"Oh?" Paul folded his arms, making the muscles bulge under the sleeves of his button-down shirt.

"Just a little work." Ryan forced a smile. He hated lying and hated being in uncomfortable situations. "Nothing major." *Except your Teacher of the Year recognition.* "Really."

"I don't get it." Paul blocked the door and leaned on the frame. "When we're on the field, I don't expect you to talk to me. We play for opposing football teams and all, but here? You can be civil and even pretend I don't have facial fungus. I don't care what colours you fly. Do you just dislike social situations or do you hate me? Tell me the truth."

Jesus. Confrontation and it wasn't even ten in the morning. As much as he'd rather have Paul's arms wrapped around him, Ryan sidestepped Paul.

"I'm just quiet and I don't like hanging around schools." Ryan pushed through the next door and allowed himself to breathe when he reached the outside. Cringing, Ryan climbed into his Jeep and rested his head on the steering wheel.

There were so many things he did want to say to Paul. *I like to talk to myself to work out problems. I have a slight obsession with art supply stores and I'm shy in public. I'm dominant in the bedroom and love using nipple clips and floggers. Oh, and I have a massive crush on you and I want to use said toys on you.* Yeah, not going to happen.

Ryan engaged the engine and backed out of the parking spot. He'd have to talk to Paul again tomorrow when the Griffins took on the Dragons for the first of their Saturday afternoon match-ups.

When he arrived back at the art building on campus, he didn't get out of his Jeep. Instead he stared at the graffiti painted on the beige wall. *Respect yourself. Love life. Live art.*

"The problem with Paul isn't that I don't like him," he said to himself. "The problem is that I do like him." The past crept up on Ryan. Flashes of his relationship with Duke came to mind. The hurt rushed back to him in waves. Being himself had cost him what he had thought was the love of his life. The pain had never really gone away, it had just sort of flatlined.

"I resolved not to fall for anyone again." Ryan sat up, but his shoulders sank. "Except I never expected to find someone like Paul and I've fucked it up."

Paul stared out of the window as Ryan ran out to the parking lot. The guy made no sense. On the field, Ryan Malone was a dynamo. His punts tended to end up on the one-yard line and his field goal attempt record was off the charts. He'd completed a fifty-four-yard field goal! So what was it about Paul that turned Ryan off?

"You're pretending to be a still life?" Laubenthal stepped between Paul and the doors. "Right?"

"Just thinking." Paul scrubbed his hand over his face then turned to the principal. "Am I that off-putting to you, George?"

"Huh?" Laubenthal raised one eyebrow. He removed his glasses and wiped them on the handkerchief he'd taken from his pocket. "Come again?"

"I'm a nice guy. I don't pick fights with people and I'm clean. What is it about me that turns people off?" Paul sighed.

"You must be talking about Mr Malone." Laubenthal placed his glasses back on his nose, then pocketed the handkerchief and clasped his hands behind his back. "Do you recall Jeannie Martin?"

"Yeah, the English teacher who only ever spoke in class. Once we got into the teachers' meetings she clammed right up." Paul snorted. "I suppose she's now a pop singer or something? Got out of the classroom and became famous?"

"No, she was extremely shy. That and very laid back. She never showed how she felt because she wanted to fly below the radar. Malone is kind of like that, don't you think? Or he's guarded until you get to know him. Something like that."

Before Paul could answer, the principal strolled away. Paul scrubbed his chin with the back of his hand. Shy? Ryan didn't strike him as a shy person. Self-absorbed and snobby fitted so much better. Nothing about Ryan should've kept him on Paul's mind. He wasn't into tall guys or lanky guys. Ryan was both. Then there were those blue eyes. The palest blue and ringed with a thin line of sapphire. The scruff on his cheeks darkened his face just a bit and Paul wanted to kiss him. He yearned to nibble his way from Ryan's chin to his lips and all over his face.

"I don't care if he's shy or that I'm crazy turned on by him," Paul muttered, then headed to his classroom. "I'll worry about him later." He counted out the pieces of paper needed for his next class. "Later."

* * * *

The next afternoon, Paul sat in the locker room at the Northwestern College recreation centre and hid his head under a towel. He hadn't slept the night before. His mind wouldn't shut off. Thoughts of Ryan and whatever bothered him crawled under Paul's skin. During the game, Paul hadn't been any better. He'd screwed up three snaps and failed to protect the quarterback twice, both times resulting in crushing sacks.

"You okay, man?" Aiden sat down next to him and tugged the towel. "You played like shit. Do I have to beat your ass or are you going to tell me what's going on?"

Jack sat down on Paul's left. "It's that kicker. I saw him watching the bench like a hawk."

The tips of Paul's ears burned and he refused to look anywhere but at the tiles on the floor.

"The kicker? The tall skinny kid who's all legs?" Aiden elbowed Paul's ribs. "You do realise he's the enemy, right?"

"And he helped score the points to put the Dragons over the top, right?" Jack groaned and stood. "Just fuck him already. Get him into your system or out of your hair. Either way, do something so you get your head back in the game. I don't like losing."

"Kiss my ass," Paul muttered. He enjoyed hanging around with both Jack and Aiden, but since they'd become a couple, they thought they knew everything about relationships.

"You don't want him kissing your ass," Aiden said. "His lips probably taste like my ass."

Paul suppressed a sigh. He knew what Jack and Aiden did when the lights went out. Descriptions weren't necessary.

"But," Aiden continued, "you're not happy. If you were, then I wouldn't have had to retrieve two snaps. Go talk to your kicker. Maybe he's into you too."

"Yeah?" Paul snapped and sat up. "He ignored me. Flat-out fucking ignored me."

"When?" Aiden folded his arms. "Do I have to kick his ass?"

"No." The fury in Paul's veins subsided. "We barely know each other and we play for opposing teams. What did I expect? Him to just fall for me? That's crazy. But I would like to talk to him. You know, get to know him. See if we're compatible. That sort of shit."

"Ouch, you've stepped out of your teacher mode and into pissed-off, slightly jealous lover mode." Aiden slapped Paul on the shoulder. "Talk to him again. Maybe he freaked out because he wasn't sure what to say. You'll never know unless you do."

Paul nodded. He hated to admit when Aiden was right and he sure as hell wasn't going to tell the quarterback. *Time to stop wallowing in my angst.* He tossed the sweaty towel into the hamper and grabbed his bag. *I'll talk to him or die trying.*

Chapter Two

The hot water sluiced over Ryan's body and took away the sting from overexerting his muscles. Eight kicks in one game wasn't his usual. But with Jason Eckles, the normal punter, out with a broken toe, Ryan had picked Jason's punts in addition to his usual point after kicks. Thankfully the Dragons had won. He had something to be happy about. They had creamed the Griffins, beating them by more than twenty points.

He turned off the spray then shook the water out of his hair. His thoughts wandered to Paul. Every time he had looked over at the Griffins' bench, Paul had sat staring in his direction. Ryan covered himself with a towel then palmed his crotch. The nice thing about being the last one in the showers was that the rest of the team had vacated the locker rooms by the time he finished. The alone time enabled him to settle down and plot out what he wanted to do for the next game.

Footsteps slapped on the concrete and the sound grew closer. Ryan poked his head out of the shower room. His breath hitched and his grip on the towel loosened. Paul Toth in the flesh...in the opposing team's locker room.

Paul tossed his bag on the floor. His eyes blazed with anger and frustration. "There you are."

"Here I am," Ryan replied. He retied the towel and hoped his erection wasn't obvious. Then again, what did he care? "You're in foreign territory."

"I get by." Paul levelled his muscle-corded shoulders. "You never answered my question."

Ryan's heartbeat hiked up and blood surged through his veins. He'd fucked things up before by succumbing to his shyness. No more letting the past get in the way of his future. Besides, talking with Paul wasn't going to lead anywhere, was it? But if it did, Ryan would take every advantage.

"I'm sorry, I didn't." Ryan stepped toe to toe with Paul. He kind of liked craving a man who stood a couple of inches taller than he did. "I don't have anything against you. You're a very sexy guy." He measured his words. "Caught me off guard when you remembered my name at the school. We don't talk much, you being on the opposing team and all. I'm glad you came in here."

"Oh." Paul's lips parted and his gaze softened. He wobbled a bit on his feet. "Thought maybe we could go for coffee."

"That's a possibility." The heat from Paul's body radiated over Ryan. He breathed in the scent of Paul, sweat and deodorant...and something pine. If Ryan bounced on his toes, he'd be able to kiss Paul.

Paul's Adam's apple bobbed. "Um..."

"Are you going to kiss me or just stand there?" Ryan assumed his role as the dominant. He didn't give Paul time to answer and captured his mouth in a kiss. Paul softened and gripped Ryan's arms. His tongue tangled with Ryan's and his cock pushed against the tent in

Ryan's towel. Ryan swallowed Paul's groan, then broke the connection.

Pink tinged Paul's cheeks and his eyelids drooped. "Whoa."

"I've got you down to one-syllable words. Nice." Ryan sidestepped Paul and opened his locker. "Guess that also answers your question." He yanked his shirt down past his head then hiked his boxer shorts past his hips.

"Can we go somewhere and talk?" Paul slumped on the bench next to Ryan.

"Yeah. I need to ice my knee." Ryan eased his jogging pants up over his boxers and unballed his socks.

"I've got ice." If it was possible for Paul's ears to turn redder, they did. He furrowed his brow and dropped his head into his hands. "God."

Ryan grinned. At least he had the man on edge. "How about we go to my place?" He could control things there much better. "Are you game to cross the line from rivals on the field to something more?"

"I'll follow you."

Ryan laced his running shoes then grabbed his bag. The fear of starting something new battled with his natural tendency to control the situation. Something about Paul felt different. Paul walked one step behind and to the left of Ryan.

"I'm at twelve-twenty Rosewood." Ryan stuck his key into the lock on his Jeep. "Meet me there?"

Paul nodded once then strode to a Mazda.

Ryan checked his mirror every once in a while to see if Paul was still behind him. His thoughts scattered. What if the whole thing was a joke? What if he'd come on too strong? What if Paul freaked the way Duke had? What if he'd made a huge mistake? He groaned.

Damn overthinking. He pulled into his driveway and parked in the garage.

"It's not the end of the world if he walks out. It's just another day." Ryan stared at himself in the rear-view mirror. "Heart's protected and thoughts in check." He climbed out of the Jeep and rounded the back of the vehicle.

Paul stuffed his hands into his pockets. "You got me here."

"I do." Ryan waved his keys. "Come on." With Paul on his heels, Ryan strolled into the kitchen. He tossed his bag on the dining room floor. "Want a bottle of water?"

"That'd be great."

Ryan grabbed two bottles from the fridge then turned around. Paul cornered him against the fridge door.

"What is it about you?" His body pressed to Ryan's, Paul's eyes widened. "You're an enigma. I feel like I know you and like I know nothing at the same time. Part of me wants to hate you because you're a Dragon. The rest of me wants to fuck you against the wall. And the other part..."

"What does it want to do? The other part?"

"To have you fuck me within an inch of my life." Paul crushed his mouth over Ryan's and ground his groin into Ryan's.

The slight push helped Ryan decide what he wanted to do. Bottles in hand, he nudged Paul back. "Do you want to play?"

"Play?" Paul's breath skittered over Ryan's cheeks. "I want to do what you want me to."

Ryan threaded his fingers with Paul's and led him to the bedroom. "Strip." He leaned on the door frame, then opened one of the bottles of water. "I want to see you. All of you."

Chest heaving, Paul grabbed the hem of his shirt and hoisted it up over his head. His nipples stuck out, dusky brown. A smattering of dark hair covered his pecs and directed Ryan's gaze to the waistband of his jogging pants. His abs flexed with every breath.

Ryan's mouth watered. He loved a well-built man and Paul had everything the way Ryan liked. "Go slow."

With a wink, Paul popped the button on his pants and kicked out of his running shoes. He fixed his gaze on Ryan and unzipped. His cock bulged from the hole in the front of his underwear. He hooked his fingers in the elastic and urged his swishy pants to the floor. Paul stroked himself through his boxer briefs then stepped out of the tangle of fabric at his feet.

Ryan suppressed the urge to fondle himself. Seeing Paul unwrap himself was present enough for the moment. He took another draw of the water.

"Like what you see?" Paul bent over long enough to shuck his socks then stood tall again. "Now what?"

"The boxers have to go." Ryan tossed the second bottle to Paul. "Have a drink." He walked around Paul's nearly nude form, taking in the beauty of the man.

"Do I measure up?" Paul touched Ryan's arm. "Do I?" He took a drink from the bottle and some of the water dribbled down his chin and slid over his chest.

"You'll do." Ryan nodded to the bed. He wanted to lick the exact spot where the droplet landed. "Ditch the boxers. I want you across my bed."

A twinkle lit up Paul's eyes. He shoved the cotton fabric to his feet then plopped onto the bed. He spread his legs wide. His cock stood proud, surrounded by a thatch of blond curls.

"You get into watching?" Paul wrapped his fingers around his erection. His sac bobbed with each stroke. "I wanted to do a little more than whack off."

"I'm observing." Ryan stepped across the room and stopped between Paul's knees.

"Tell me what you want me to do." Paul scooted to the edge of the bed.

"You know what I want you to do." Ryan rested his hands on his hips. His cock pressed tight against his jogging pants.

Paul peered up at Ryan and smoothed both hands under Ryan's shirt. Ryan blew out a long breath and kept his groan quiet. Paul flicked Ryan's nipples. Heat rolled through Ryan's body. He rocked his hips. "That's good. More."

Without breaking eye contact, Paul bunched Ryan's shirt, then helped him remove the garment. Paul gasped. He latched onto one of Ryan's nipples. Electricity shocked Ryan's system and centred in his groin. His balls tingled. Ryan threaded his fingers in Paul's short hair.

"Now work on the other one." Ryan nudged Paul.

Paul released his hold then kissed his way across Ryan's chest. He toyed with the nipple he had abandoned with one hand and gripped the waistband of Ryan's pants with the other.

"Yes," Ryan panted. He shivered as the cool air swirled around his dick. Paul let go of Ryan's nipple with a pop, then kissed his way down Ryan's abdomen to his cock. He flicked his tongue across the blunt head of Ryan's erection, lapping up the bead of pre-cum. Paul's groan turned Ryan's senses inside out.

"Fuck." Ryan fisted his hands in Paul's hair and ground his teeth. "Take me in."

"Yes, sir." Paul opened his mouth wide and took Ryan to the back of his throat. He hummed and massaged Ryan's erection with his tongue.

Ryan grunted and set the pace, fucking Paul's mouth. His belly flip-flopped and power surged through his veins. Hearing Paul call him sir brought back good memories. He preferred to be in control, and with Paul, he could be. Paul's natural submissive tendencies needed to be brought more fully to the forefront.

Paul smoothed his fingers up and down Ryan's hips, stroking his body. He continued to hum and work his mouth over Ryan's cock.

"Stop." Ryan held himself in check. He didn't want to go off so soon. "Lie down for me."

Once again, Paul gazed up at Ryan. He smiled around Ryan's erection then released him. He stretched out on Ryan's bed and grinned. "You're going to use that on me?"

"So eager." Ryan grabbed a bottle of lube and a condom from his dresser. "I should make you wait." He tore the condom package open. "Should make you put this on me, too."

Paul sat up and took the rubber from Ryan's hands. He rolled the condom up Ryan's cock then nabbed the lube.

"You're pushy." Paul squirted lube on his hand and Ryan's dick. The contact, even through the latex, seared Ryan. Paul was a quick study if he wasn't already playing submissive games. The more they played, the more Ryan wanted another encounter with the dark-haired centre.

"You like it." Paul collapsed on the bed, knees in the air and a wide grin on his face.

Ryan lined up his dick with the tight ring of muscle in Paul's hole, then pushed. Paul's eyes widened for a moment and more colour rushed into his cheeks. He moaned and grasped Ryan's arms.

"Shit." Paul writhed on Ryan's cock. "I'm full."

"More short sentences. Good." Ryan pushed balls deep into Paul's ass and embraced the desire coursing through his body. Paul relaxed around him and met him thrust for thrust. *Time to take things up another notch,* Ryan decided. He situated Paul's legs around his waist, then crawled onto the bed. He leant forward, pinning Paul's arms above his head with one hand.

"Oh fuck," Paul panted. "Yeah."

Ryan rested his forehead on Paul's then pinched Paul's nipple. "You'd look so hot in handcuffs, all stretched out for my perusal. Nipple rings on your nipples gleaming in the light and a cock ring around that massive wood. Like a beautiful statue and all for me."

"Yeah?" Paul replied. He swiped his tongue across Ryan's bottom lip. "Tell me more."

More? Holy shit, yeah. Ryan pumped harder. The combination of Paul surrounding him and the dirty talk heightened the oncoming orgasm. He didn't want to come so soon, but fuck, with such a sexy man turned on by Ryan's kinks, Ryan couldn't hold back.

"Your ass needs a paddling, too. I can see it now, your butt so red and hot and just for me." Ryan let go of Paul's nipple, then stroked his cock. "Come for me. Show me how hot I'm making you."

"Ryan." Paul trembled and his legs quaked. He shot his load in twin ribbons on Ryan's chest. His breathing stuttered and he fought Ryan's grasp. "Fuck."

Pleased with Paul's response, Ryan surged one last time into Paul and filled the condom. His balls ached from holding in the orgasm so long. He released his grip on Paul's wrists and braced himself on his hands.

A bead of sweat trickled between his shoulder blades and he puffed to catch his breath.

"We really crossed a line, didn't we?" Paul smoothed a perspiration-soaked strand of hair from Ryan's eyes.

Ryan opened his mouth to say something, but his phone rang from the other room and interrupted him. He shook his head. He'd worry about the phone later.

"You should get that," Paul said. "Might be important."

"And ruin the post-sex glow?" Ryan pulled out of Paul then stood. He tossed the spent condom in the garbage.

"I'll still be here when you get back." Paul settled against the blankets. "Don't think I could move if I wanted to."

Ryan snagged his boxers from the floor. "I'll just be a moment." He growled under his breath and left the bedroom. He knew the ringtone — his ex, Duke.

"What else could go wrong?" he grumbled to himself and pressed the buttons to answer the call. "What the hell else?"

Chapter Three

Paul stared at the ceiling. A solid fuck by a Dragon. Well, shit. He'd intended to go into the locker room to talk—not play tongue hockey with Ryan. Hadn't planned on the kiss and had never dreamt he'd follow Ryan Malone home. Now he lay in the middle of Ryan's bed after mind-blowing sex.

Unreal.

Ryan had left the room and, wherever he was in the house, Paul couldn't make out what he said. The tone spoke volumes. Whoever the caller was, Ryan wasn't thrilled.

Paul sat up and glanced around the room. He needed to get dressed and go. He doubted Ryan had expected the call, but the things he was saying to whoever was on the other end were pretty damned intense.

Within a few moments, Paul had dressed and laced his running shoes.

"Hold the fuck on." Ryan stomped into the room. "I'm sorry."

"No big deal." Paul shrugged. He hiked his bag onto his shoulder. "I'm out of here."

Ryan placed his hand over the cellphone receiver. "Hold on." He moved his hand. "It's over. You said no, so no it is." He punched the buttons with his index finger then tossed the phone on the bed. "I'm sorry."

"You said that."

"*That* wasn't supposed to happen." Ryan forked his fingers into his hair. "Asshole."

"Ex?"

"He dropped me then conveniently forgot what he'd done." Ryan dropped his hands. "It's messy, but it's over."

"Gotcha." Paul nodded. "I'm out. Papers to grade and a dog to feed. Zeppelin gets cranky when he thinks he's being neglected."

"Here." Ryan scribbled something on a piece of paper. "Call me?"

"You got it." Paul dipped his head once. When Ryan tugged his shirt and pulled him close for a kiss, Paul didn't resist. He sighed and tangled their tongues. Kissing Ryan was easy. Hell, doing everything he'd done with Ryan had been too easy.

Ryan swirled his tongue over Paul's bottom lip, then severed the connection. "Call me."

"I will." Paul panted and wobbled his way to the door. His thoughts jumbled and he barely noticed the drive home. He pulled into his driveway then stopped in the garage. While the garage door shut, he gathered his wits.

Ryan was the enemy, part of the other team, and one of the few men, other than Aiden, he wasn't supposed to sleep with. But he couldn't get Ryan out of his head. The guy kissed like a champ and his attitude—no one ever told Paul what to do, except Aiden and Jack, not even the coaches or the medical staff. They gave him a wide berth. And no one pushed him around like Ryan. Still, whatever was drawing them together was strong.

He tossed his keys and wallet on the counter, then checked his email on his phone. His dog trotted into the kitchen and plopped down at his feet.

"Hiya, girl." He petted Zeppelin's head then fed her. He sorted through his bag, separating out the dirty clothes while she ate. When he had finished, she followed him to the bedroom, where he flopped on his bed with his laptop. The dog hopped up beside him. The Siberian husky stretched out and swished her thick tail. A tuft of black and white fur flew in the air and landed on his keyboard. She groaned then stretched again.

"Thanks, Zep. You shed everywhere. Jeez." Paul tossed the wad of fur into the wastebasket then pulled the search engine up. "Who are you, Ryan Malone?" He entered Ryan's name into Google. More than likely he wouldn't find anything. "God, I don't want to be a cyber stalker." He looked away from the screen, hoping nothing came back in the results. When he turned his attention to the screen, three hundred results had come back.

"Holy fuck." Paul frowned and clicked on the first link. *Kicker leaves NFL after punishing tackle.* NFL? Like the National Football League? No fucking way. He scanned through the article. "He played pro?" He scrolled down the page to the image. Ryan lay flopped on the field, his left leg turned at an odd angle. The injury looked like hell. He continued reading. *Malone's recovery expected, but his return to the game doubtful... After three years of rehab and practice, Malone regained full use of his leg as well as most of his talent. He's settled down to a quiet life in the art world.*

"Shit." Paul stretched his hand out and patted Zeppelin's head, more for his own moral support. "No wonder all the teams wanted him. He's a ringer and a freaking former celebrity." He closed the lid of the computer. No wonder Ryan didn't talk much. God only knew what kind of crazy followed him around. People liked to associate with celebrity. Did Ryan deal with that? Or was he so full of himself he thought he was better than everyone else? Somehow that didn't seem fitting. Ryan didn't drive a flashy car or have women crowding the locker room doors, waiting for him. Ryan was just Ryan.

Zeppelin whimpered and stretched out. She flopped her tail on the bedspread twice then settled.

"Are you thinking about Ryan, too?" Paul placed the computer on the nightstand then yanked his shirt up over his head. "I'll call him later, girl. Right now I'm beat." He settled beneath the covers. Two hours before, he had lain stretched across Ryan's bed. Paul closed his eyes. Being with Ryan had worn him out, body and soul. For a change, he welcomed the feeling.

* * * *

Paul adjusted his shoulder pads. The last week hadn't gone as planned. Every time he had picked up his phone to call Ryan, something else had gone wrong and grabbed his attention. He'd forgotten the end of the term and the onslaught of projects he had to grade. Then there was the incident at the vet's office with Zep. The dog hated going to the vet, but she'd never taken so long to come around after the sedatives. Paul was prepared to have the vet come to the house, regardless of the cost, if it meant keeping her safe and healthy.

Aiden strolled up next to him and handed him his jersey. "So."

"So." Paul ducked his head and worked the jersey over his pads.

"You talked to him, didn't you?" Aiden folded his arms. His helmet swung from his fingers. "The kicker."

"Yes." Although he told Aiden just about everything, the encounter with Ryan wasn't on the to-be-discussed list. Paul sat down to put his socks on.

"Details?" Aiden waggled his fingers. "Did you two do the nasty?"

"Enough." Paul's ears burned and he focused on lacing his cleats to ignore his embarrassment. "It's not up for debate. You can tease me all you want, but yeah, we talked."

"Talked." Aiden snorted and sauntered off.

Paul blew out a long breath and finished his last-minute padding adjustments. If he moved his ass, he'd be able to catch the last few minutes of the Dragons' game versus the Phoenixes. He hurried out of the locker room to the field, then checked the scoreboard.

Fifty-five seconds left with the Dragons down by two. Paul clutched his helmet in one hand and clapped his free hand against his thigh. Ryan stood on the forty-yard line practising kicks.

The article came to mind. According to the picture, Ryan kicked with his left foot. The practice kicks were being done with his right foot. *Wicked devil*, Paul thought. *Ambidextrous. Nice.*

The whistle blew and Ryan backed away from the player who would hold the ball once the play started. The quarterback hiked the ball back to the holder, who placed it for Ryan.

Paul bunched his hand. "Through the uprights," he murmured. "Do what you're good at."

Ryan connected with the ball, kicking it right in the middle of the uprights. At the same time, the line wavered and two players made it through. Both men, larger than Ryan, dived into him and tossed him to the ground. Ryan's head snapped back, striking the field first. Whistles blew and two yellow flags soared through the air.

The wind rushed from Paul's lungs. He hadn't been with Ryan long, if they were even a couple, but seeing the poor man crushed under the defensive ends made Paul's stomach churn.

"Get up, buddy," Paul chanted. "Get up." He balled his hands and zoned in on Ryan. The longer Ryan lay stretched out, the farther Paul's stomach fell. He didn't belong on the playing field, but he wanted to rush out there and check on his lover—no, friend. He growled to himself. They had to figure out what the hell they were to each other. He wanted more than friendship or a casual fuck.

More whistles blew. The coach and the med students rushed onto the field. Paul couldn't see over the mass of people crowding around Ryan.

"Make it, man. Don't let this shit happen twice," Paul murmured. "Someone get out there and check him. Damn fool could be concussed."

"He'll be okay." Aiden bumped Paul's shoulder. "He might be the enemy, but I don't want to see him hurt. He'll be up in a moment and I'm sure they'll run a concussion test on him. That was a bad hit."

"He played pro." Paul searched the crowd for Ryan. "Got hurt this way and ended his career."

"The hell you say," Aiden replied. "Looks like he's up. You planning on getting him up later?" Aiden jabbed his elbow into Paul's ribs. "You'd better be if you haven't planned on it already. But be careful. If his noggin's fucked up, you'll both be up shit creek without a paddle."

Go figure Aiden would be a punk and say something so ridiculous, even if he was right. Paul focused on Ryan again. With the help of a med student and one of the coaches, Ryan made his way off the field. He wasn't putting much weight on his left foot.

Paul strode forward to talk to Ryan, but Aiden held him back.

"Seriously?" Paul brushed Aiden off. "You say stupid shit, but don't want me to check on him? Blow off."

"Don't start with me." Aiden grabbed Paul's arm and hauled him away from the sideline. "He's hurt. Yeah, you two have a thing, but right now he's being checked over. After our game you can do whatever you want with him. He'll be fine until we're done. We need you."

Well, fuck. Aiden was right and damn him for being so. Paul put on his helmet and shook his head. "Get in the game," he chanted. "Get in the game."

The match-up between the Griffins and the Hydras went by in a blur. Paul held the line and tackled harder than he had intended. After seeing what had happened to Ryan, Paul wanted blood. When he stood in the locker room afterwards, he thought more about Ryan. He cared about the kicker, more than he probably should've. They had shared one afternoon of sex. Was it passion? Maybe. Was it the best sex he'd had in a while? The best ever. No matter how hard he tried, he couldn't get Ryan off his mind.

"Why don't you go check on him?" Aiden handed Paul his gym bag. "He's the enemy, but he's a hot enemy."

"I thought I was the only person you thought was hot." Jack slung his arm around Aiden. "You're not looking again, are you?"

"You're such a dork." Aiden winked. "Let's go, sexy." He and Jack walked off, hand in hand.

Paul zipped his bag and closed the locker. He wanted what Jack and Aiden had. Wanted that love to last forever and the same smile to wake up to in the morning, like they shared. He needed the same man in his arms. Someone stable and honest. Someone to love him.

Who was he kidding? He wanted Ryan in his arms. Screw the phone call. He'd visit Ryan in person.

After a twenty-minute drive across town to Ryan's neighbourhood, Paul stood at his front door. Maple trees with their leaves beginning their fall switch from green to bright yellow towered along the street. Fingers of orange late day sunlight stretched down the worn pavement and glittered off the row of two-storey homes. A couple of the houses featured white picket fences surrounding the front yards. The trickle of water from the fountain in front of the house reminded Paul he needed to go to the bathroom. The weight of the day combined with the chill in the air and brought out a shiver from deep in his bones.

He pressed the bell and waited. A wave of embarrassment washed over him. Ryan would not be able to answer the door. Not with a busted leg.

The door budged and a short woman with shoulder-length blonde hair grinned. Her green eyes sparkled. At her full height, she barely reached his shoulder. "Can I help you?"

"I'm here to see Ryan." Paul fidgeted with his keys. If he hadn't been gay, she might have turned his head. "He's not expecting me. Is he feeling up to company?"

"You're not Duke, are you?" She narrowed her eyes and her eyebrows bunched. "Are you?"

"Duke? No, I'm Paul Toth. We play football together." Kind of. Paul scrubbed the back of his neck with the palm of his hand. "Thought I'd check on him."

"Good, and he'll appreciate it." She opened the door wider. "Come in. Ryan's on the couch." She waved her hand and ushered Paul into the living room. "You have a visitor who isn't Duke the Dud."

"Chrissy." Ryan massaged his forehead. "Hey, Paul." Thick bandaging wound around his right leg.

"I'll leave you two alone. I've got…a…bun in the oven," the blonde stammered. She wagged her hand in the air then pointed at Ryan. "Yeah. A bun."

"Chrissy, do you have something to tell me?" As he shifted on the couch, Ryan's face paled. "Or something you're not telling me?"

A blush swept across her cheeks. "No."

"Then don't say a bun, unless you're pregnant." Ryan held out his hand. "Thanks for staying with me. I'll call if I need you."

"You'd better." She kissed his temple, but her blush deepened. "And tell me the details." She winked at Paul then sashayed out of the room.

"She's my neighbour." Ryan shrugged. "She's sweet, but not my type." He grinned. "The week I moved in, she showed up with a cherry pie and offered to let me sample both."

Paul settled in the nearby chair. "And you told her…you weren't interested?"

"I was blunt. Told her I was gay and although I love cherry pie, hers didn't do anything for me. Once we accepted each other's differences, we became friends. It's good."

Paul shifted in his seat. He wanted to ask what had happened, but the walking cast spoke quiet volumes.

"Nathan Korrs didn't hold the line and the two biggest Phoenix players broke through. I paid the price. It's not broken, but I couldn't put weight on it.

Doctors put the Ace bandages on so I wouldn't move it too much. I'll have to do physical therapy to get it back in shape, but I'll get past it." Ryan shrugged again. "Not much fun to be around, am I?"

"You're fine." Paul reached for Ryan's hand. "You'd be surprised." An idea popped into his mind. "You know, even if you can't move, I can."

"Going to give me a show?"

"Perfect idea." Paul stood and pulled his phone from his pocket. He'd never danced for someone, but for some crazy reason he wanted to entertain Ryan. The guy looked so depressed. Paul pressed the buttons for the first song he came to. KISS. Nice. "Watch me."

Ryan tipped his head, but didn't move. Hunger and something else, something like desire, shone in his eyes. Paul shifted his hips and grabbed the hem of his shirt. His pants swished with each movement. He kicked out of his shoes, then inched the bottom of his T-shirt up on his chest. Ryan nodded and clapped his hands. Paul worked with the rhythm and removed his shirt. He tossed the garment across the room, then turned around, giving Ryan a view of his ass.

Behind him, Ryan groaned. "Show me more."

Oh yeah. Paul eased the jogging pants down his ass, keeping his junk covered. He wiggled his butt. "Better?"

"Come here." Ryan grabbed the back of the pants and pulled Paul to his side. He rubbed his nose along Paul's hip. "Fuck. Bend over."

Paul yanked the coffee table close and planted his hands on the oak top. He waved his butt. "What are you going to do to me?"

Ryan shoved the pants the rest of the way to the floor and spread Paul's ass cheeks. Hot breath swept over his hole, followed by the hot swipe of Ryan's tongue on Paul's skin. Paul groaned. Jesus. Ryan pushed his tongue into Paul.

"Damn." Paul backed into Ryan and rolled his hips. He didn't want to have all the fun. Hell, Ryan was the hurt one. As much as he loved being rimmed, Paul stood and focused his attention on getting out of his pants. He kicked the tangle of clothing to the side then dropped to his knees.

Paul moved Ryan's shirt out of the way and kissed his abs. He licked the salt on Ryan's skin and groaned as Ryan tugged on his hair. Paul kissed his way up to Ryan's nipples, taking extra care to touch most of Ryan's chest.

"God, that feels good." Ryan tightened his fingers, pulling the strands of hair at the back of Paul's head. "Shit."

Paul dragged his teeth over Ryan's nipple. "Move your hips." He curled his fingers in the elastic waistband of Ryan's shorts.

"You like being pushy?" Ryan asked with a chuckle.

"Only while you're hurt." Paul rose up and braced one hand on the back of the couch. He wrapped his other arm around Ryan's neck and decided to follow his heart. "I'd rather you be in control."

Chapter Four

He'd rather me be in control? Cool. Ryan stared at Paul. He understood his partner enough to know what he wanted, but he'd never expected to hear the words out loud.

Paul kissed Ryan's cheeks, chin then his nose. "I'm a natural follower. I like you leading." He punctuated his sentence with nips on Ryan's lips. "Now I'm going to take care of you until you get better and can spank my ass." He bobbed his eyebrows. "You want to and I want you to."

"I do." Ryan spread his hands on the cushion then rose up enough for Paul to ease the shorts down his thighs. Once Paul wrapped his fingers around Ryan's cock, Ryan sat forward and kissed Paul again. "Can't get enough of you."

Ryan hadn't planned on confessing something so private, but the harder he tried to hold back, the more the words tumbled from his lips. "Want this."

Paul nodded then flattened his tongue across the blunt head of Ryan's cock. Sizzles started in the base of his dick and surged to his balls. After the shit from the game, the pain of his injury, being with Paul and being pampered by Paul hit the spot. Paul licked along the underside of Ryan's cock, drawing a groan from deep in his throat. He reached down between Paul's legs and caressed his dick.

"Fuck," Paul said around Ryan's erection. He then took Ryan to the back of his throat and swallowed, massaging Ryan.

Ryan shifted to keep his left foot elevated, while still stroking Paul. He winced and his breath caught. Paul stopped licking Ryan's dick and tipped his head to meet Ryan's gaze. Ryan's cock popped out of Paul's mouth, shiny with saliva.

"You okay?" Paul trailed his fingers over Ryan's temple, then down his jaw.

"Just aches. My leg." The concern in Paul's voice tripped Ryan up. The more time he spent with Paul, the more he cared about the man. He wanted to possess Paul, not just fuck him every once in a while.

"You're sure? I don't want to hurt you." He kissed Ryan again. "Never thought I'd say this, but whatever this is between us isn't just a fling." Paul stared at Ryan for a moment then resumed sucking Ryan's cock.

Ryan threaded his fingers in Paul's hair. No matter how hard he tried, he couldn't get Paul's revelation out of his head. Not just a fling? They'd only fucked and talked for a short period of time. Sure, he'd stared at Paul's picture while he had completed the painting, but Paul didn't know anything about the work of art...did he?

Paul dragged his teeth down Ryan's cock, bringing him out of his thoughts. "Oh, shit," Ryan gasped. He wriggled his hips, pumping in and out of Paul's mouth. He groaned. Nothing else mattered. In that moment, the rest of the world faded away and the only thing Ryan noticed was Paul. Fever rushed through his veins and he released his grasp on Paul. He clawed the couch cushions and gritted his teeth. The orgasm came on too strong, too fast.

"Holy fuck," he groaned. "Fuck." Ryan surged deep into Paul's mouth and shot his load down Paul's throat. He puffed to catch his breath. From his head to his toes, he couldn't move.

Paul sat back on his heels and licked his lips. "Feel better?"

"Feel like I'm floating." Ryan's head lolled on his shoulders. He watched Paul from under heavy eyelids. "Good, though."

"Yeah, you're good to me, too." Paul spread his hand across Ryan's stomach. "I came without hands on me. That's never happened." He grinned. "I loved it."

Ryan suppressed the wince. His leg ached. Part of him wanted to be scared and hide away from the feelings blossoming in his chest. The rest of him wanted to embrace them and Paul. He wasn't Duke and the sword of fame didn't hang over his head any longer. Besides, Paul hadn't asked about Ryan's life before coming to town. All that mattered was the present. Only time would tell if things between them would go awry, but if he didn't try, he'd never know.

"Good thing I have another shirt in my bag." Paul laughed and his shoulders bobbed. "I came on the one I was wearing."

Ryan gave in to the infectious laughter, but sobered. "Stay." His heart beat faster and his palms itched. He wasn't ready to say love, not after two encounters, but he wanted Paul to stick around.

"I'd love to, but I've got to let the dog out."

"Oh." Ryan nodded once. "No problem."

"Mind if I bring Zep over here? Next time? She's good about not chewing on things, plus you can meet her. She likes other men, but women aren't her thing. She's very protective of me around women." Paul dug through his bag and withdrew a fresh shirt. "I'd love to talk art with you. Most of the guys I know don't know their Rivera from their Mondrian."

"Two totally different styles."

"Exactly. Plus I'd love to learn about the restoration side of the museum. Fascinates me how you can take a painting that's assumed to look one way, scrape off the grime and it's a totally fresh, explosive work again. I'd probably try to fix it. Change the parts that don't work for me. Guess I'm more of a control freak than I thought."

"Nothing wrong with knowing what you like." Ryan hiked his shorts up and shifted into a sitting up position. "Restoration is painstaking, but worth it."

Paul finished dressing. "Can I call you when I get home? I'm not sure I want this to end, but you're in no shape to go anywhere."

"Why don't you bring her over tonight?" Ryan shoved his shaking hands under his thighs. He couldn't remember the last time he'd asked a lover to stick around, much less bring their dog over. "I don't want things to end either and I've always wanted a dog." Not totally the truth, but not a total lie either.

"Yeah?" Paul left his bag on the floor and bunched his wallet and phone in his fist. His keys jangled. "Give me half an hour and I'll be back." He leaned in for a kiss. "I love you." He nipped Ryan on the lips then bounded out of the room.

I love you? Ryan settled in the pillow and massaged his temples. Love meant complication. Complication meant his heart wasn't safe any longer. Then there was the dog... *I'm in a relationship. For the first time in a long, long time, I'm not alone. Holy shit.*

* * * *

Paul clicked the leash onto Zeppelin's collar and walked her out to his Mazda. "Come, girl. We're going for a ride."

The dog raced past him and climbed into the back seat. Instead of sitting, she paced and panted, leaving wet spots on the leather. Any other time he'd care. Not when he knew he'd be spending more time with Ryan. He started across town and talked to the dog.

"I've never met anyone like him, Zep." He glanced in the mirror at her. The dog finally sat down. "Good girl." Paul turned onto Ryan's street. "I'm not relationship material, but every time I'm around him all I can think of is spending more time with him. Like forever time. It's nuts. Promise me you won't act up."

Paul parked in Ryan's driveway and helped the dog out of the car. "Remember, Zep, be nice." He grabbed the extra overnight bag and the dog's supplies from the trunk.

Footsteps slapped on the concrete behind him. "I hoped I'd catch you."

He recognised the voice. Chrissy. "Hi. Thought I'd bring the dog back and keep Ryan company tonight."

Chrissy offered her hand for the dog to sniff. "You're a pretty girl, aren't you?" When Zep finished checking out Chrissy, she snorted and sat down next to her. "She's well-behaved, too."

"I trained her well. Unless I'm in harm's way, she's fairly docile."

"Good." Chrissy glanced up at Paul. "He's been through the wringer. I'm sure Ryan doesn't want me to talk about it, but he's my friend and I'm kind of like

the dog. If you fuck with him, I'll fuck you over, too."
She stood at her full height, up to Paul's shoulder. "I
don't know who Duke was, but he ran Ryan through
the mud. Ryan played professional ball, yeah, but he's
not some dumb jock. He's smart and funny and when
you get past his barriers, he'll love you deeper than
you can imagine."

"I hope he does." Paul gripped the leash tighter. Not
because he thought something would happen to Zep,
but because he hadn't expected Ryan's life to be so
bumpy.

"Well, good." Chrissy folded her arms. "I expected
more of an argument from you."

He shrugged. "I don't like to argue."

"Just—don't break his heart. Okay? Don't." She
unfolded her arms and wagged her finger at him. "I
will hurt you if you do."

"I'd expect you to." Paul whistled. "Come on, Zep.
Chrissy, thank you. I'll take good care of him and feel
free to keep an eye on the both of us."

"Okay." She smiled and strolled down the sidewalk
to her house.

The dog whined and danced at Paul's feet. "We're
going in."

"I think she sees me." Ryan limped towards Paul.
"Wondered if you got cold feet."

"Nope. Waylaid by your neighbour." Paul offered
his free arm. "Don't overdo it. You'll fall and need
more than an MRI."

"I won't argue with you. It hurts too much to bitch."
Ryan hobbled next to Paul as they made their way to
the front door. At the steps, Ryan took extra time. "Go
ahead."

Paul opened the door and unhooked Zeppelin's
leash. "In and sit." The dog whipped past him and
tore into the house. "Dogs."

Ryan chuckled. "As long as she doesn't leave a bomb or a puddle, I don't mind." He gripped the railing and hopped up the last step. "Jesus. I hate being hurt."

"You just about had your leg ripped off in a play. You can be hurt." Paul escorted Ryan back to the couch. "You want here or on the bed? Where's more comfortable for you?"

"The bed. I can get there." Ryan bumped Paul's shoulder. "But thanks."

The house wasn't large and Paul remembered the way to the bedroom. He slapped his thigh. "Zep."

The dog trotted to his feet and sat down. "Get Ryan. Make friends with him." When Zeppelin took off down the hallway, Paul made sure to click the fob on his keys to lock the car then grabbed his extra bag. He strode to the bedroom. Zeppelin hadn't made noise and, knowing her as he did, silence couldn't mean good things.

"You're a pretty girl, aren't you?" Ryan sat up on the bed and scratched Zep behind the ears. If Paul didn't know better, he'd have thought they'd always been together. He grinned. Another sign he and Ryan had something fantastic going between them.

"I'm going to fill her dish and get her some water. Do you need ice?"

Ryan's cheeks flooded with colour. "Yes. You don't have to."

Paul leaned on the door frame. "Hey, I'm cool with exploring you being in control in the bedroom. But right now, you're hurt. I'm all for taking care of you. Let me do it."

"Okay." Ryan resumed talking to the dog.

Minutes later Paul settled next to Ryan on the bed. Zeppelin stretched out on the edge of the bed and commenced snoring.

"Wish I had bought a dog." Ryan nodded to Zep. "She's good company."

"Speaking of company..." Paul shifted and threaded his fingers with Ryan's. "About what Chrissy said."

"She's good at being overprotective." Ryan didn't look at him.

"I agree. She's also good at threats. She mentioned someone breaking your heart and that you weren't famous, so I shouldn't expect you to act like it." He pressed his lips together. He'd added a bit to what she'd said, but he didn't care. "I know some of your past. Google is a wealth of info."

"You Googled me?" Ryan frowned. "I'm still on there?"

"You are." Paul cupped Ryan's chin. "And sexy as hell in those jerseys." He rubbed his thumb along Ryan's bottom lip. "Look, I know you went pro. I don't care. I've got a life and I'm happy with it. I'm attracted to you, not the celebrity. Even if you never play again, my feelings won't change. Crazy, since it's not been very long since I crossed the line and made a play for you. But my guts aren't wrong and my guts say this is something that was meant to happen."

"I'm glad you're so confident." Ryan squirmed. "She's right, though. Duke claimed one thing then did something else." He sighed. "If you want to be with me, there's a few things you need to know. I play hard when I fuck. Normally I'm not hurt and skittish. I take control. I'll push you places you never thought you'd go, but I'll never fuck you up. But before we start anything like that, I mean, really hardcore stuff like spanking or my tying you up, you have to accept it. I won't force you, but if you have any doubts, tell me now."

Paul parsed through what Ryan had said. He'd never played 'hardcore' and he wasn't about to do something just to convince a man they had chemistry. But the idea of having his ass paddled intrigued him. The bondage part sounded kinky and fun, too. Knowing Ryan the way he did and banking on Ryan's honesty, he believed Ryan would never do anything to intentionally hurt him or fuck him over.

"How about you rest and once you get the green light to fool around, we'll explore? I want to, but I don't want you to screw up your knee more than it's already screwed up."

"Cool." Ryan leaned over and retrieved a book from the floor. "You mentioned Mondrian. Thought I'd share the latest show at the gallery." Ryan handed Paul the book. "This is my artwork. These are the parts of me I don't usually share with people, but I'm sharing them with you."

Chapter Five

Paul flipped through the book, taking the time to look at each photograph. The paintings included sports images as well as imagery of people. What really caught his eye was the amount of gore and blood in Ryan's work. More than a couple of the paintings had bodies with holes where the heart should've been. He touched the image of a lone figure curled in a ball and surrounded by blue. The work reminded him of a joyous Matisse gone wrong.

"That's *Forlorn*. I struggled through it." Ryan tried to turn the page.

"What did Duke do? I can see his hand all over that painting. He might not have painted it, but I feel your pain in it like it was my own. It makes me ache."

"Really?" Ryan's gaze vacillated between the book and Paul. "You see all that? Huh." He rubbed his chin. "Duke and I were together for two years. Over the first year, I denied who I was in order to make him happy. He wanted someone who didn't demand in bed. He wanted two minutes with the lights out and only on Thursdays. Sad but true. Maybe not the Thursdays part, but you get the idea."

"Vanilla to the extreme?"

"And I'm not." Ryan shifted the ice on his knee. "I like things to have a hard edge. When I played for the Browns, I ran with a fast crowd. After I got hurt, I came out and accepted who I was. I liked control and I enjoyed playing with a submissive who could handle being controlled. I explained all that to Duke. He first saw the dollar signs, which meant shit to me. I banked a bunch back, but my first love is art. I live off what I make at the museum. Then he decided he wanted to try playing the way I wanted to play. He found my crop and a ball gag I had and wanted to use them. So we did. For the second year of our relationship, I thought we had something good."

"But you were wrong?"

"He was good at hiding. Poker face good."

"So the more you tried to read him, the more he hid. Nice."

"Sucked. I watched so carefully and thought I understood his needs. I was so wrong. He shook my confidence in myself and my ability to love someone else. If he'd just talked to me—"

"Then we wouldn't be here right now." Paul stroked Ryan's cheek. "I've never played a bondage game. I've seen things, but never indulged. If I feel like I can't handle it, I'll tell you. I don't play poker very well and I wear my heart on my sleeve. What you see is what you get from me."

"That I can handle." Ryan yawned. "I haven't had anyone stay over since him, so if I'm out of practice, you know why."

"Let's sleep. If you need me, you know where I am." Paul picked up the melted bag of ice and carried it to the kitchen. He dumped the water and turned the bag inside out to dry. The more he learned about Ryan, the more he liked him. Maybe there was danger in getting too close too fast, but he didn't care. He welcomed whatever Ryan wanted to throw at him.

* * * *

Ryan sat on the crinkly paper at the doctor's office on the examination table and groaned. The swelling had gone down after two days and the bruises had finally faded. Having Paul there for the last week had helped. He wasn't keen on relying on Paul and hated feeling so needy.

The door creaked and Dr Rasmussen ambled into the room. "Good afternoon, Ryan. I have the results of the MRI." He sat down on the stool and flipped open a folder. "You're thirty-three and this is your second major sprain on your left knee."

"I'm a kicker. Normally I don't get tackled. This time I got pummelled." Ryan twined his fingers together. "I'm done, aren't I?"

Dr Rasmussen sighed. He closed the chart and folded his arms. The stool clicked as he leant back a bit. "It's not good. You can't afford to keep tearing the ligaments and expect to continue playing at the current level. You're not old and you're in excellent shape, but I'm concerned that one more injury will impair your ability to walk."

"Jesus." He could live without football, but walking? Shit.

"I don't think you're going to let the injury get that far. So, yes, I'm suggesting you give up the Saturday league. Maybe you could coach or work at the college with the special teams. But your kicking, even as a hobby, is done."

Ryan nodded. "How long will I have to do PT?"

"Six weeks and you'll be fine. Otherwise your knee has bounced back and I'm glad. I'm impressed. Every time you get hurt, you bounce right back. Just don't overdo it."

"Can I finish the season? We've got two games left."

"But the Dragons are headed for the interleague play-offs and you're not just place kicking, you're the punter as well."

"Got it. I'm done."

"In addition to the healed-over sprains, you're developing arthritis. Too much overexertion and you'll regret it."

"Got it."

Dr Rasmussen filled out the paperwork. "This is your order for PT. I don't want you to end your career, but I'd like you to think about hanging up your cleats."

Ryan folded the papers and paid his co-pay, then headed to the outpatient area of the hospital. Once he had set up the times for his therapy, he sat in his Jeep and called Paul.

"Do you have a moment?" Ryan couldn't keep the frustration from his voice.

"My lunch period starts in ten. Come in and we'll eat in my room."

"You're sure?"

"Why not? I don't care that my co-workers know I have a boyfriend. Might be a good role model for the students. Meet me in ten in the office."

Fifteen minutes later, Ryan stood in the high school foyer and waited on Paul. Windows leading to a glassed-in courtyard allowed ample light into the building. The occasional black tile broke up the monotonous white tile leading down the hallways. Trophy cases overflowing with the fruits of the school's sports teams' labour lined two walls. Ribbons for swimming, football helmets and photographs of the athletes filled the spaces.

"There's my guy." Paul's smile lit up his eyes. "I'm glad you're here. My room is at the other end of the building." He escorted Ryan past countless nondescript tan doors leading to other classrooms. They turned down a hallway lined with artwork. One whole wall featured the sea life in a pond. Ryan grinned. Nice to know Paul mixed art and science in his lessons. When they reached the black and white door to the art room, Paul ushered him inside then closed the door. "I usually leave it open, but I'd like privacy. So what's up? You had your appointment today." He turned his chipped maroon chair around backwards and sat down at one of the large wooden desks.

"I'm done." Ryan sat down hard on the closest chair. "Done."

"With?"

"Football. One more sprain and my knee is shot. Done. So, I'm benched for the rest of the season. I've been benched before, but I always thought I could play for fun. Now I can't do that."

"Do you live and breathe football?"

"No. I'm an artist. Football was my stress release."

"Then embrace what you love." Paul opened the baggie with his sandwich. "PB and J. My favourite." He broke the sandwich in two. "Have some?"

Ryan took the jagged half offered. "I never expected to have to totally give up the game."

Paul chewed and didn't say anything for a long time. "I've never been hurt so badly that I couldn't play. But I'm the centre. I take hard hits. Being on special teams, you're not expected to get roughed up." He took another bite, waiting until he finished chewing to continue. "It's not like you have to give up everything. You can probably play touch football in the backyard. Kick a few just for fun."

"You're right."

"Whether you can play or not doesn't faze me." Paul shrugged. "As long as you're not totally avoiding the game, I'm happy." He checked his watch. "Speaking of happy, I only have five minutes before twenty-three sixteen-year-olds come charging in here. I wanted to tell you something that I couldn't say in a text."

"Okay." Ryan bit into his half of the sandwich to keep from saying something really foolish.

"I've been thinking about what you said when we" — Paul glanced around the room — "made love the last time. I want to try whatever you can throw at me."

Ryan coughed, nearly choking on the sandwich. He patted his chest. "You do?"

"Yeah." Paul grabbed Ryan's hand. "Ease me into it, but I've been dying to try this. I've even got a list of things I know I don't want to do." He grinned. "I wanted to ask you something else."

"Shoot."

"The seventh is the awards banquet for the faculty. I'd like you to come with me."

"What if things don't work out? What if we play" — Ryan dropped his voice to a whisper — "and you decide you don't like to play the games?"

"Duke shot your confidence to hell, didn't he?"

"Yeah."

"I can't help you get back into football and I don't really want to if it means you'll get hurt, but I'm more than willing to help you regain your confidence." Behind Paul, the bell signalled the end of the period. "And that's my cue to walk you out."

Paul escorted Ryan back to the office. "I'll call you after school. I've got practice tonight, but think about what I said." He hesitated for a heartbeat then kissed Ryan on the lips. "Love you."

Winking, Paul walked backwards into the foyer doors, then pivoted and headed into the building.

Ryan drove back to his office and considered what Paul had said. His confidence was shot. Duke leaving had torn a hole in his heart and scarred his soul. Then had come Paul. He wanted to help Ryan become the man he'd been.

For three straight hours, Ryan mended the tears and frayed edges of two pages of a Book of Hours. He had damn near cried when the museum had purchased the collection of pages and cherished his time with the delicate relics. He also planned out what he wanted to do with Paul.

On the way home, Ryan stopped at his favourite place to shop. If he couldn't find the toys he wanted at Heaven, he wouldn't find them. He waved at Callie then shopped for what he wanted. Their first time needed to be intense, but not so over the top that Paul would run screaming into the night. He placed his items on the counter.

"You finally found someone?" Callie rang up the toys and handcuffs. "I'm proud."

"It's a possibility." Ryan paid for the merchandise. "Time will tell."

"Fingers crossed." She held both hands in the air. "Good luck!"

"Thanks." Ryan left Heaven and set out for home. He turned the radio on and sang along with the songs to keep his thoughts off what he'd planned. Excitement surged through his veins and he drummed on the steering wheel. Maybe he had found the someone he'd been waiting for. Maybe.

Chapter Six

Ryan arranged the items on the dresser. His hands shook and butterflies filled his stomach. He tapped his foot to the song playing in his head. Ten more minutes and Paul would arrive.

"Ryan?" Footsteps clunked on the hardwood floor in the kitchen. The scratch of Zeppelin's nails echoed in the quiet house. Paul peeked around the corner, but Zeppelin barged right in and took her place on the bed. She swished her tail and panted.

"Hiya, Zep." Ryan patted the dog's head. "Pretty girl."

"She was excited to get here." Paul snagged Ryan in his arms. "So was I." He stopped moving. "We get to use all that?" He touched the end of the crop.

"Second thoughts?"

"Not a one." Paul trailed his fingers over the butt plug. "I'm intrigued, yes. Scared? A little. Wanting to do this? More than ever."

"Cool." Ryan patted the bed. "I have something for you, Zep." He grabbed the rawhide from the grocery bag. "This is for you."

The dog jumped off the bed and nabbed the bone from Ryan. She settled on the rug and gnawed on the knotted end of the treat.

"You took the phrase 'love me, love my dog' to the extreme. She'll never want to leave," Paul whispered in Ryan's ear. "I like the way you think."

"Zep?" Ryan clapped his hands. "Out here for now." He strode into the guest bedroom. "Over here." He patted the bed. "All yours until we're done."

The dog hopped onto the bed and resumed working on the bone. Ryan headed back to the bedroom. "I'll leave the door open."

Paul settled on his knees. "Ready, sir."

"What are the rules?" Ryan picked up the crop. "And what is your safe word?" He slapped the flat end against his palm.

"Cougar." Paul bowed his head. "I don't wish to use the word but if I do, I'll tell you because you expect me to speak."

"Good." Ryan swatted his palm again. This time the sound ricocheted off the walls. "Couple more things. Give me the list of what you won't do."

Paul tipped his head. "Needles, blood, knives, because I saw that shit and it kind of scared me."

"It's intense and not something I do." Ryan opened his hand on the back of Paul's neck, stroking his hair. "Anything else?"

"I don't want anything attached to my face or tongue."

"Wax?"

Paul looked up at Ryan. "Maybe. I've never tried it, so I'll give it a shot."

"Blindfolds?" Ryan continued to stroke the back of Paul's neck, learning his lover.

"Bring 'em on." Paul grinned. "I'll give those ball gags a shot, too. But they won't work if you want my mouth on you." He licked his lips. "I can be very persuasive."

"You can." Ryan kissed Paul's forehead. "If you decide something else is on the not-going-to-happen list, tell me. As much as I'm in control, you control what we do or don't do."

"I understand and wish to play, sir." Paul dipped his head. "I'm yours."

"Yes, you are." Ryan folded his arms. "Stand and undress. Slowly. Show me what I'm waiting for."

Without making eye contact, Paul stood. He kicked out of his running shoes then shrugged out of his shirt. The garment landed on his gym bag. He rolled his shoulders, giving Ryan a delicious view of his toned body. Ryan dragged the flat end of the crop down Paul's spine.

"Ever thought about getting a tattoo?" Ryan tapped the crop on Paul's shoulder blade. "Right here."

"I have, sir." Paul hooked his fingers in the waistband of his pants. "I know what it would be, too."

"Really?" Ryan rubbed circles over Paul's skin with the leather end of the crop. "What?"

"A paint palette with two brushes." Paul shoved the jogging pants to the floor. "And something else." He straightened up and his cock tented his boxer shorts.

"What else?" Ryan circled around Paul, stopping behind his lover to grab Paul's ass. "What else?"

"Our initials."

No hesitation. Ryan massaged Paul's ass cheek. "I see."

Goose pimples rose on Paul's skin. He kicked his pants and socks to the pile. Instead of shucking his boxer shorts, he stood still.

"You're not naked." Ryan slapped Paul's ass with the crop. "You want to be punished?"

"Yes, sir. Thank you, sir." Paul glanced over his shoulder. "I deserve punishment."

"Naughty." Ryan swatted him three more times on each cheek. "Drop the boxers."

Paul eased the fabric over his cock then the boxer shorts settled at his feet.

"Good." Ryan tapped Paul's ass with the flat of his hand. "I love how your butt turns so pretty and red." He twirled the crop in his fingers. "Now how should I dole out your punishment?"

"Spank me, sir?" Paul clasped his hands behind his back. "I'm yours to do with whatever you want."

"You are." Ryan slapped the inside of Paul's thigh with the crop. The sound echoed. "Spread your feet."

Paul widened his stance.

"Nice." Ryan tucked the crop under his arm then took the set of handcuffs from the bureau top. He clicked the cuffs around Paul's wrists. The scent of sweat and desire hung heavy in the air. A bead of perspiration slid between Paul's shoulder blades. Ryan breathed him in and dragged his tongue over the patch of skin where he'd suggested Paul have the tattoo added.

"Thank you, sir," Paul moaned. He flexed his fingers. "May I have some more, sir?"

"Not yet." Ryan imagined the tattoo emblazoned on Paul's shoulder blade. Their initials… The idea wrapped tight around Ryan's brain. The more he considered it, the more he liked it. "Lean over the bed."

Paul shuffled to the mattress and bent at the waist. He waved his ass proudly in the air. This time, Paul watched Ryan's every move.

Ryan traced his fingers over the three plugs he'd purchased. Paul wasn't ready for the larger plug. Not yet. He selected the medium-sized plug, a vivid blue one with a set of ball bearings embedded in the plastic.

"Who do you belong to?" Ryan nabbed the bottle of lube then slicked the plug by running his fingers over the toy's smooth surface. His own cock responded and bobbed between his legs.

"I belong to you," Paul responded. "Let me take care of you, sir."

"In a moment." Ryan stroked the plug once more then pressed the thinner end against the tight rosette of Paul's ass.

Paul groaned and bore down on the toy. The blue plastic disappeared in his hole, stopped only by the thick lip at the base of the plug.

"Thank you, sir." Paul rolled his hips. "Damn."

"You like it?" Ryan stepped back then gripped the crop. "You're getting too comfortable with the plug." He slapped the backs of Paul's thighs. "How many times should I punish you?"

"Thank you, sir. More." Paul shivered.

Ryan reached between Paul's legs and arranged his cock so that it pointed to the floor. "Can't let you get yourself off on my comforter." He resumed spanking Paul, tapping circles over Paul's butt. The skin turned a delicate shade of pink. Paul unclenched his hands, but the muscles in his legs tightened.

"More?" Ryan swatted him again, starting at the top of Paul's bottom and moving down to the backs of his thighs. He slapped thirteen times, making sure to touch every inch of Paul's butt.

"Thank you, Sir." Paul groaned again. "Feels good."

"Good." Ryan tucked the crop back under his arm. He waited a moment and debated his next move. Power surged through his veins and love filled his mind. God. He'd become more attached to Paul than he'd figured. He smoothed the leather end of the crop over Paul's balls. "Should I touch you here?"

"I'm yours," Paul replied. "You may touch wherever you want."

Ryan opened his palm on Paul's ass. He tapped the plug with his thumb.

"Oh shit." Paul bucked off the bed. His legs trembled and his movements turned jerky. "Fuck."

"Touched something special?" Ryan twisted the plug then tapped it again. "No coming until I tell you to."

"Yes, sir." The words came out tight.

Ryan grinned. He kept the crop in his fingers, but backed away from Paul. "Stand."

Paul hesitated a moment. Without his hands to help him lever his body off the bed, he lost some of his grace. He rose to his full height then bowed his head.

"You need something else to make you pretty." Ryan ran the chain of the nipple clamps through the fingers of his other hand. "These." He offered the chain to Paul. "Do you like?"

"Thank you, sir. I like them a lot."

Ryan twirled the crop then held it before Paul. "Open. Bite." When Paul bit down on the shaft of the crop, Ryan palmed Paul's pec. He rolled Paul's nipple, then sucked on the dusky flesh. Beneath Ryan's mouth, Paul shivered. Ryan bit Paul's nipple, taking extra care to scrape his teeth over the sensitive skin.

"Sir," Paul said around the crop then bucked again. Pre-cum glistened on the tip of his cock.

Ryan affixed the first clamp on Paul's nipple. "So pretty." He gave Paul's other nipple the same treatment then attached the second clip. The chain glittered in the light and swung slightly. He removed the crop from Paul's mouth then tugged the chain. "Bite."

Paul's eyes widened, but he complied. The clips pulled his nipples up, stretching his skin.

"Do you wish to use your safe word?" Ryan caressed Paul's cheek. "Do you?"

Paul shook his head. "No, sir. Thank you, sir." He wobbled on his feet and his eyelids drooped. Tiny whimpers and sighs escaped his lips around the chain.

"Beautiful." Ryan trailed his fingers down Paul's chest. Seeing his lover drifting into subspace turned him on and turned his senses inside out. He loved how Paul responded to each push.

"One more thing," Ryan murmured. He turned the cock ring over in his fingers. With Paul already hard, the original ring he'd picked wouldn't fit. He opened the tiny hinge in the ring then wrapped the steel circle around Paul's cock and balls.

"Jesus," Paul gasped. He dropped the chain.

Ryan stared at Paul. "You may use your safe word if you'd like."

"No." Paul opened his mouth. Ryan replaced the chain between Paul's lips.

"You're sure?"

Paul nodded. "Feels like fucking heaven."

Ryan folded his arms. What to do next? He twirled the crop again then swatted Paul's stomach. Paul winced and groaned, but didn't back away. More pre-cum leaked from his cock. He puffed each breath and his head lolled on his shoulders, pulling the chain tighter.

"Fuck. Need to be inside you." Ryan took the chain from Paul's mouth then turned him around. He wriggled out of his shirt and tossed the garment out of sight. His pants ended up in a heap at his feet. "So fucking hot, I don't want to wait."

Ryan caressed his cock, pulling and stroking himself. His balls tingled and flutters started in his belly. He groaned.

Paul planted his face on the blankets and waved his ass. "Fill me, sir. Make me feel every inch of you."

"What do you say?" Ryan slapped Paul's ass. He nudged the toy, caressing Paul's prostate.

"Thank you, sir." The muscles in Paul's back writhed and tightened. "Take me, sir. I'm yours. Fill my ass and take me. Please, sir."

Begging… Ryan's one weakness. He loved to hear his lover plead for orgasm. He twisted the plug, removing it from Paul's stretched hole.

"Thank you, sir," Paul answered.

Ryan tossed the used toy onto the pile of clothes then grabbed a condom from the bureau top. He sheathed himself in one swift move. As much as Paul wanted him in his ass, Ryan couldn't wait any longer to take Paul. He lined the blunt head of his cock up with Paul's asshole then pushed past the tight pink skin. Inch by inch, Paul took Ryan in and squeezed around him.

Shit. The tingles from his oncoming orgasm took over too damn fast. Ryan grabbed Paul's hips and went from thrusting to pistoning in a hot minute. His body quaked in time with Paul's trembles. Both men groaned. Ryan slammed into Paul, his balls slapping on Paul's sac.

"Fuck." Ryan's growl ripped through the room and he dug his fingers into Paul. He'd tried to hold back, but no longer. The dam burst and the orgasm took over. He pumped seed into the condom then slouched over Paul. His vision blurred and his knees wobbled.

"Sir." Paul's pleading tone pulled Ryan from his post-sex haze. He rolled off Paul then released the cuffs. He helped Paul onto his back.

Ryan climbed astride Paul's thighs and unhooked the cock ring. "Stroke yourself. I want to see you come." He stayed in his place on Paul's lap and took in the sight of Paul masturbating himself.

Paul used both hands to stroke his cock. Within a moment, a thick rope of cum splattered on Paul's chest. Another ribbon of cum splashed on Ryan's chest. Paul sagged on the bed and gasped for breath. Sweat glistened on his chest.

"Let me remove these." Ryan loosened the clips on Paul's nipples then kissed the abused skin. He stretched out atop Paul. "You're so fucking hot when you come."

"Yeah?" Paul stared up at him from under his lashes. "You're hot, too. Thank you, sir."

"Sleep." Ryan kissed Paul on the lips. "Rest and let me clean you up."

Paul nodded and continued to stare in the direction of the ceiling. "Lost my breath." He waved his hand. "I'll clean me up."

"You're good." Ryan placed both of Paul's hands on his chest then climbed out of bed. He opened the door a bit more and patted his thigh. "Zep."

The dog jumped off the bed, bone in her mouth, and trotted back to Ryan's bedroom. Ryan strode to the bathroom and ran a washcloth through hot water. He caught a glimpse of himself in the mirror. The glow had returned. Instead of the sallow, sad man he usually stared at, a happy man had taken his place. He cleaned the drying cum off his chest then grinned at himself. He liked the improved mood. Sexy did look hot on him. He squished the water out of the cloth then returned to Paul.

Eyes closed, Paul hadn't moved. Ryan rubbed the damp cloth over Paul's cock and chest, cleaning him.

"Thanks." Paul rolled onto his side. "Love you." He sat up, scrubbed both hands over his face then wobbled to the bathroom. When he returned, he curled up on the right side of the bed.

Ryan hung the cloth on the rack in the bathroom then settled beside Paul in his bed. He and Paul fitted together so well, like they'd been lovers forever. Ryan let his guard down and closed his eyes. "I'm pretty fond of you, too."

* * * *

Paul spent the next two hours in and out of sleep. He scrubbed both hands over his face, then watched Ryan sleep. The relationship was so fragile, so new, but the things they'd done...holy shit. Paul should've been scared. Grown men spanking other grown men. Some people might not think a simple spanking was bad, but...damn. Or the clips, the butt plug and the other things... Jesus.

His body ached all over, but nothing he'd trade. Each sting reminded him of what he had shared with Ryan and brought to mind moments of their play. He touched his tender nipples and whimpered. The pain felt too damn good.

The dog padded next to the bed and sat next to Paul. She bumped his hand with her head. Even in the moonlight, he could see the yellow glow in her eyes.

"It's okay," he whispered. If things were okay, why didn't he feel so okay about it? He groaned. The whole idea of seeing Ryan was to talk things through, not fall into bed after one meeting. They were supposed to have sex without feelings—except he'd added the feelings and Ryan had added the pinch of chains and spankings. Part of Paul felt ashamed for what they'd done. Part of him was even more intrigued and ready to play a second round. Ryan pushed the limits, but he talked during the sexual activities. He didn't shout or belittle Paul. No, the whole experience came off quite loving and safe, despite the handcuffs and clips.

His brain buzzed. Too many thoughts and no way to shut them off. If he didn't crash soon, he'd never make it through the next day. Screw it. He needed to walk off the energy coursing through his veins and sort his thoughts out.

Paul inched out of bed and gathered his clothes. He patted his thigh to signal to the dog to follow then headed into the hallway to dress. The less noise he made, the better Ryan would continue to sleep. Once he had dressed and rounded up the items for the dog, Paul led Zeppelin out to his car. Embarrassment and regret crashed through him. Duke had fucked Ryan over after a scene and what was he doing? Walking away, just like the ex. Except he wasn't going away for good. No, he needed time to process.

He scribbled a note then ran back into the house. Not the best way to ask for a temporary break, but then he'd never been so head over heels before.

Zeppelin whimpered and wiggled on the passenger seat.

"We'll be back." He put the car in gear. "I promise. I'll make things up to him and we'll work it out. Once I digest what happened. I just need time to think."

Now if Ryan would understand...he'd be golden.

Chapter Seven

Ryan rolled over and opened his hand. Instead of touching warm male, he touched cool pillow. The temperature change jerked him awake. He sat up and glanced around the room. No clothes on the floor, no dog, nothing. His heart sank.

"This had better not have happened to me again," he muttered and climbed out of bed. He pulled on a pair of boxers and shuffled through the house. A note lay on the kitchen counter.

Sometimes a man has to think. I need to think. Give me some time.

Ryan crunched the paper in his hand. Time. They always wanted time. He massaged his temple. Well, if Paul wanted a break then he'd get one.

Although he wasn't focused on his work, Ryan navigated through two days at the museum without calling Paul. On the third day, he picked up his phone but didn't dial. What was the use?

He resumed cleaning a set of coins from Greece and attempted to push Paul from his mind. While he scrubbed, his phone rang.

"Hello?" Ryan propped the phone between his shoulder and his ear while he dried his hands.

"Hey."

He knew the voice. Paul. Ryan closed his eyes to keep the onslaught of frustration at bay. He kept his voice level. "You left."

"I did."

"Want to tell me why?" Ryan's voice cracked, but he kept calm.

"I'm not comfortable."

"I see," he bit out. *Fucking shit.* Ryan's emotions hit with full force as the past reared its head. *Don't let your aggravation win out,* he reminded himself. *Let him explain...if he can.*

"You see?" Paul's voice dropped to a whisper. "Really?"

"Really." Ryan sat down hard on the closest stool. For as much as the past hurt, he wanted the present and future with Paul so much more. "Yes. You got it. Got into what we did, and because you liked it, you freaked. The whole idea of being spanked was a turn-on until it happened and you liked it more than you expected to. Your brain screams it's not a good thing, while your body craves it. Then I did the other things to you and those turned you on more. It takes time to process all those good feelings and understand it wasn't done to shame you, but to set you free."

"Yeah."

"Remember how you told me not to give into the depression Duke caused? You were going to help me win my battle. Well, the same goes for you. Don't back away from what we have because of fear. Yes, part of what we did is considered fucked up by normal folks, but tell me, who in the hell is all that normal?"

"True."

Ryan's heart beat triple time and he drummed his fingers on the desk to calm down. "I found my confidence. If you can't handle what I am and how I play, then fine. Tell me so we can do what we have to do. If you can handle it, you know where I am."

"Ryan."

"I'm not arguing with you. I'm done fighting for the right to be myself." Ryan clicked the button to disconnect the call. As much as his chest ached at the possibility that he'd lost Paul, strength buoyed him. He'd finally stood up for himself and accepted who he was.

"Hooray for me." Ryan placed the silent phone on the desk then picked up another soiled coin. "I've got scars and shit in my closet I don't want to share, but I am who I am."

His phone rang again, but this time he knew the ringtone. "I need to delete that damn tone and number." Ryan declined the call, but before he could walk away, a text popped up.

Rybear need 2 see U.

Miss U.

Rybear. Shit. He'd hated that pet name from the moment Duke had come up with it. Ryan deleted the texts then removed Duke's name and number from his phone. He didn't want the hassle or the reminder of past mistakes. "He dumped me. Now I'm dumping him for good. Enough with men who don't know what they want and expect me to sort it out for them." He tossed the phone back onto his desk. "I've got bigger things to deal with."

* * * *

Paul stared at the silent phone. Ryan had done the last thing he had expected. Hung up on him. The nerve. The whole point of the call was to settle things, not tear whatever kind of relationship they had to smithereens.

He only had himself to blame. Everything Ryan had said made perfect sense. The things they'd done were consensual and had turned Paul on. He did crave the next encounter. Craved having Ryan's arms around him and his breath on his skin. Memories of the sting from the crop filled his brain. He liked being filled with the plug and giving himself up to what Ryan wanted to do, even if he actually controlled the actions.

Paul shoved the phone across his desk and forked his hands into his hair. He stared at the wrinkled blotter on his desk. Each day since he'd gone into the locker to room to talk with Ryan he'd marked the days off on the calendar. Twenty-six days. Could life change in twenty-six days? For him, life had turned completely upside down.

"Mr Toth." Laubenthal ambled up to Paul's desk. "Something on your mind?"

"No." Paul sat up straight and rested his chin in his hand. "What can I do for you? My evals aren't until next week. Was there a scheduling issue? You're welcome to come into my classroom at any time for the evaluations."

"Oh, there's no issue." The principal handed Paul an envelope. "The itinerary for the award ceremony. We'll have you do some lettering like you did last year. Are you bringing a date?"

"Uh…" Paul glanced over the paperwork. He didn't see his name next to any of the categories. "I don't know. Thought about begging off this year. If I'm not nominated, there's no point in going."

"You don't want to do that. You love seeing the winner with the painting. "

"I didn't do it this year."

"Oh, that's right." George rubbed his chin. "Ryan Malone did." He waggled his finger. "Very nice job he did, too." Without looking at Paul, the principal strolled out of the room.

Ryan had done the painting? Well, no wonder he'd been hanging around the school. Why hadn't he said anything? Paul would've loved to have given him perspective on what the painting should've looked like. They could've spent even more time together.

Hell. Spent time. They should've been together for the past three nights, not arguing on the phone and avoiding each other. Screw it.

The moment school recessed for the day, Paul jogged out to his car. He sped across town to the museum. He'd soul-searched enough and didn't care what others thought. The sex rated somewhere in the stratosphere. If Ryan wanted submission, then Paul would give it.

He parked at the back of the museum next to Ryan's Jeep then strode around the building to the main doors.

The woman at the main desk smiled. "May I help you?"

"I'm here to see Ryan Malone. He doesn't know I'm here. I wanted to surprise him."

"Oh." She picked up the phone and pressed buttons. "Yes, I have a visitor. Send him back? He'll need a pass, unless you'd rather not see him." She shuffled some papers. "Okay, I'll do that."

"Well?"

"He says no." She folded her hands. "He's very busy on a set of Greek coins and can't be disturbed."

"I see." Paul ground his teeth together. Things weren't happening according to his mishmash plan. He tipped his head to the woman then sighed. He might as well take a look at the new acquisitions exhibit. He stuffed his hands in his pockets and appraised the prayer trunk. Six hundred years of abuse and neglect showed on the piece, despite the cleaning. Next to the trunk sat a pair of manacles, engraved and inlaid with jewels.

"Bizarre," Paul murmured. The handcuffs glimmered under the bright lights. "Who would make them look so beautiful and why?"

"They belonged to someone very wealthy." Ryan's reflection smiled beside Paul's. "Thought I'd find you here."

"I quit hiding." Paul glanced at the cuffs. "Someone wealthy or with a kinky streak?"

"Probably both." Ryan folded his arms and matched Paul's stance. "You wanted to talk."

"Not out here."

"I wanted to show you something." Ryan turned on his heel and strode away from Paul. "Keep up or Marjorie will think you're trespassing."

Whatever. Paul hustled to keep up with Ryan. Together, they navigated a set of corridors to what Paul guessed was the back of the building. "Where are we?"

"My office." Ryan produced a set of keys and unlocked his door. "Wait." He lowered his gaze. "There are certain things about me I don't share. With anyone. When I played pro, there were all these people wanting something from me. They expected my life and my money would make them better somehow. I never set out to get rich and I don't like huge crowds. I wasn't smart enough to find someone worthy of sharing my life with back then."

"And now?"

"I shared my need for kink with you. You saw the inner part of me no one ever sees." Ryan shrugged.

"Now I want to show you my office." He opened the door. "You can ask anyone. I never bring people back here. Ever."

Paul crossed the threshold and gasped. Three large easels took up one wall. A desk cluttered with papers and books sat in a corner. In the middle of the room, a light table shone and coins glittered. What caught Paul's attention were the easels. One had photographs taped to it, but no canvas. He crept across the space.

"Those are me." Paul ripped one of the images from the easel. "What the hell?"

Ryan didn't say anything.

"Why do you have these?" Paul tore down another photograph. "If you'd asked, I might have given you one. This looks creepy."

"Want to stuff a sock in it?" Ryan leaned against the light table. "I have those because of the painting."

"What painting?" Paul spat.

"Your Teacher of the Year painting, dumb ass. You were so hell-bent on kicking my ass for something you knew shit about. Now you know my secret. I painted your portrait. Asshole."

"Mine?"

"Come on."

Paul stopped short. He hadn't been asked to complete the painting...because he'd won the award? He wobbled on his feet. "Wait."

"Yeah. You figured it out." Ryan stepped toe to toe with Paul. "I couldn't tell you because it was supposed to be a secret. But yeah, I stared at you and thought you were hot. I wanted to meet you, but you being one of the Griffins and always up Aiden's ass, I never bothered. Did I fall for you by looking at you? Yes. Even more when we fucked? You bet. I let you into my secret, sacred world and you freaked. I'm giving you another chance and you call me a creep.

Gee, sounds like the start of something fucking wonderful."

"Ryan."

"Fuck you." Ryan closed his eyes and growled. "Just fuck you."

Paul tossed the photographs to the floor. "Yeah, fuck me." He twisted the lock on the door. "Right now."

"What the hell?" Ryan's eyes narrowed. "Don't dick with my head."

Paul stalked across the expanse of the room then cornered Ryan against the light table. "I screwed up. I said I wasn't going to fall in love and I did. Blurted it out right away, too. Then, you're right, I freaked. I'm not making the same mistake. Yeah, you overwhelmed me, but I liked it. You were right all along. I need, I crave your brand of kink." He crushed Ryan on the desk top and captured Ryan's mouth in a kiss. He ground his cock on Ryan's thigh. When Paul rocked Ryan, his ass caught on the switch. The light flickered with every movement.

Ryan gripped Paul's arms, but didn't shove him away. "We do this my way."

"Yeah," Paul panted. "I'm yours." He'd dreamt of this moment and begged for it. As long as Ryan called the shots, he owned Paul all the way to his soul. "Always."

"I see." Ryan crooked one eyebrow then shook his head once. "Plus, I don't want to have to explain how the light table shorted out." He angled Paul to his desk then swiped his hand across the surface, shoving his papers all over the floor. "On your knees."

Paul did as told and grinned up at Ryan. He loved playing the submissive, and accepted it more and more as they played. "Thank you, sir. May I taste you, sir?"

"Good boy." Ryan threaded his fingers into Paul's short hair. The tug burned his scalp. "Can't really have a scene the way I want."

"Order me, sir."

"Nice." Heat flashed in Ryan's eyes. "Take care of me."

Paul unbuckled Ryan's belt, then popped the button on Ryan's pants. He pressed his face into Ryan's trouser-covered crotch. The sweet aroma of Ryan's erection kicked Paul's desire up another notch. He unzipped Ryan then shoved both hands into Ryan's pants, pushing the fabric to the floor. Ryan's boxer shorts ended up on top of his trousers.

Seeing Ryan's beautiful erection bob before his eyes sent shivers down Paul's spine. Ryan gripped Paul's head, bringing him back to reality. "You know what to do."

"Yes, sir." Paul opened his mouth wide and took Ryan down his throat. He swallowed, massaging the blunt head of Ryan's cock. He closed his eyes and lost himself in the moment and sheer bliss of sucking on Ryan.

Ryan panted and shifted his hips. "Oh God," he whispered. "Gotta stay quiet."

Someone could probably hear them, but Paul didn't care. He grabbed Ryan's ass with one hand and stroked his balls with the other. When Paul opened his eyes, he noticed Ryan's head lolling on his shoulders. Fucking awesome. If he kept teasing Ryan, he'd blow his wad in seconds. Ryan moaned and jammed his cock in Paul's mouth.

"Umm," Paul hummed around Ryan's erection. When Ryan withdrew, Paul licked his lips. "Like honey or candy." He buried his nose in Ryan's pubes and swirled his tongue around Ryan's dick. "Could suck on you forever." The scent of Ryan stuck fast in his brain.

"Feels good, doesn't it?" Ryan traced the seam of Paul's lips, leaving a trail of pre-cum on his face. "Yeah?"

"Yes, sir. More, sir." Paul basked in the pleasure. He wanted Ryan to mark him even more. Paul moved his hand from Ryan's ass to his asshole and tapped the tight ring of muscle. "Come for me, sir. Come on me if you want. I'm yours. Mark me."

Ryan growled and tipped his head back. He breathed hard and bit down on his bottom lip muffling the sound. He grabbed the back of Paul's head, taking over the pace. "Fuck," Ryan muttered and pumped his cock in Paul's mouth. "Coming." His control snapped and his seed spilled down Paul's throat.

When Ryan came, the rest of the world faded away. The only thing, the only person who mattered was Ryan. Nothing could replace what they shared. Paul didn't want anything to replace Ryan.

Ryan gripped the edge of the desk and eased into a sitting position. His legs wobbled and his hand trembled. "Damn."

Paul sat back on his feet and wiped his mouth with the back of his hand. "Sit down." He offered his hand. "With me."

"Yeah." Ryan slid off the edge of the desk and into Paul's arms. "Can't get my bearings. It's crazy and...wow."

"You're pretty wow, too." Paul rested his head on Ryan's shoulder and wrapped his arms around his lover. The storm between them seemed to have passed. Time to put his heart on the line again. "Can I ask you something?"

"Anything."

"Come to the game this weekend." Paul stroked Ryan's bare thigh. "Please? We're playing the Minotaurs. I want you to be there."

"You're needy." Ryan took a deep breath, then kissed Paul's temple.

"You know it."

"This is nuts. Half an hour ago, I never wanted to see you again. Now I'm not sure I want you to go." Ryan sighed. He kissed Paul again on the temple, but this time the kiss lingered. "Never thought I'd christen the office like this."

"I like to offer unique and exciting experiences to my lovers." The moment he'd finished speaking, Paul realised the blunder in his words. "I mean... I wanted to make this special for you."

"You did." Ryan tensed. "About the game, I'll see what I can do."

"You better." Things weren't perfect between them, but damn it, Paul wasn't about to let a good thing slip away because he'd used the wrong words. He'd set their relationship back on track or die trying. "I'll be waiting."

Chapter Eight

I can't believe I'm doing this. Ryan climbed out of his Jeep then hit the lock. He stuffed his hands into his coat pockets and wandered to the practice fields. He'd spent the better part of the morning at the banquet hall helping to prepare the room for the awards ceremony. He'd arranged enough streamers to last him a lifetime. Granted, the school district lacked financial resources, but streamers? Jeez.

He rested on the fence and scanned the scoreboard. Five minutes to go in the fourth quarter. At least he had arrived in time to watch some of the game. He gripped the chain links and searched the sidelines for Paul. Aiden pointed at Paul then said something Ryan couldn't make out. Another man joined the fray and the three of them spoke to each other. From the bits and pieces Ryan picked up from reading their lips, none of the three were too pleased. He checked the scoreboard again. No wonder all three were pissed off. The Griffins were down by a touchdown.

"You've got time to make it up," Ryan murmured.

Paul stopped arguing and tossed the towel he'd kept around his neck. Anger radiated off him. Even across the field, Ryan noticed the wild fury in Paul's eyes.

"Focus on the game, man." Ryan took the first available seat in the bleachers. He rubbed his hands together and continued to watch Paul. The quarterback resumed practice tosses. Paul strode over and grabbed the ball. He took a three-point stance and, with the quarterback, practised snaps.

Within moments, the Griffins intercepted the ball and number eighty-eight returned the ball for forty yards.

"That gets you back towards your goal line," Ryan said to himself. He clapped as Paul and the rest of the offence ran onto the field.

Paul trotted to the huddle then stopped. He stared in the direction of the crowd. Ryan couldn't see his facial reaction, but Paul nodded a couple of times then joined the huddle.

Three snaps later, the Griffins lined up on the five-yard line. Ryan squeezed his hands together tight and bounced his knee. "Come on, guys." He pressed his knuckles to his lips. *Do what you do best.*

The quarterback took the ball and dropped back ten yards. Two players from the opposing team raced after him. He cocked his arm and threw. The pass sailed through the air towards the end zone. One of the Griffins reached towards the sky and grabbed the ball.

"Both feet in," Ryan whispered. "Please have both feet in."

The official whistled and signalled the outcome of the play.

"Touchdown!" Ryan leapt out of his seat and pumped his fists in the air. "Yeah."

The quarterback jumped on Paul, knocking him to the ground. Ryan took his seat and clapped. "Proud of you," he shouted, knowing Paul couldn't hear him. "Now make the extra point." He glanced at the clock. Less than a minute left. The Griffins had used up the clock more than he'd figured. "Don't screw this up."

The team lined up again, with the kicker set up behind the centre. The kicker completed two practice kicks then the rest of the players spread out on the line.

Paul shouted something Ryan couldn't hear and the players shuffled around the field. Three receivers lined up to one side. Instead of the regular player who held the ball, the quarterback knelt for the snap.

"They're going for two," Ryan whispered. He clasped his hands in front of his mouth and prayed. "Just make it."

More shouting this time, but Ryan couldn't tell who the noise came from. The players jumped into motion. One receiver ran straight up the middle and another one ran out wide to the right. The kicker strode forward and kicked, but at the same time, Aiden stood. He threw the ball to the receiver standing alone in the middle of the end zone. The official in the end zone called the catch fair and the crowd erupted in cheers.

"Holy shit, yeah!" Ryan jumped up and down. He bounded from his spot in the bleachers, down to the fence. If he hurried, he'd make it around the field to where Paul was. Ryan stopped by the end zone to take in the view of the next play. The Minotaur offence scurried around the field, but the Griffin defensive end batted the ball down. On the next play, the quarterback handed the ball off to the running back, but instead of making a large gain he tripped over another Minotaur player. Ryan checked the clock.

Nine seconds to go.

He laced his fingers together on the edge of the fence. Once he saw Paul, he'd give his man the love he deserved. Ryan's heart thudded. *Love*. Yes, he loved Paul more than he realised and wasn't afraid to tell anyone. The fear didn't bother him any longer. If Paul wanted to leave, then fine, but at least Ryan could look back and know he'd been true to himself. He sprinted around the field. The crowd erupted in cheers and both teams ran out onto the playing field. Paul held his helmet in the air and shouted at full volume. He turned around and opened his arms.

"Ryan?" Paul sprinted to where Ryan stood. "You came." He scooped Ryan into his embrace and whipped him around. "Didn't expect to see you here."

"Yeah," Ryan gasped. Paul squashed Ryan in his grasp. "I made it." He coughed, then Paul set him on his feet. "Proud of you."

Paul kept quiet for a long moment. "I'm sorry I ran out on you. Sorry I screwed up and didn't try to make things better right away. I didn't mean to fuck things up, but I'm in over my head. You — we're so close and I like you more than I should. Don't give up on me because I'm making a mess of what we could have."

"We all have our moments." Ryan grabbed Paul's hand. "And once you're done changing and whatever, we'll celebrate the win and what we are to each other."

"We will?" Paul's eyes widened. He yanked Ryan back into his embrace. "Damn right we'll celebrate." He kissed Ryan hard on the lips. "Don't want to wait."

"It's cool." Ryan laughed. His chest ached from being crushed, but he loved the attention. "We've got all night."

"No." Paul sobered. "The banquet is tonight."

Ryan cupped Paul's jaw in both hands. "How about you get cleaned up, gather your things and come over. You can submit to me for the rest of the afternoon then we'll shower and go to the banquet. I can't wait to show you off."

* * * *

Paul rushed through his shower and changing. He'd listened to the coach after the game, but had only heard about half the words. The only person who mattered was Ryan. Paul sped across town and excitement coursed through his veins. *His submission.* Truer, sexier words had never been spoken. Whatever Ryan wanted, he'd get. Not to make him happy, but because Paul craved the freedom of being in Ryan's bonds.

He ignored the cat calls and hoots from Aiden and Jack. Let them say what they wanted. He loved Ryan without a doubt.

After retrieving Zeppelin, Paul pulled into Ryan's driveway. Arriving at Ryan's felt like coming home. Strange and exciting at the same time.

"Hey, you." Ryan leaned on the porch railing. "You're not here for me, are you?"

The dog bounded across the yard and jumped on Ryan. She knocked him backwards onto the bench alongside the short end of the porch.

"I told you she likes you." Paul shifted his bag on his shoulder. "Me too."

Ryan nudged Zep off his lap and followed Paul into the house. "Good plays today. The Griffins are really on the mark."

"We had our asses handed to us last week." Paul dropped the bag on the nearest chair then draped his suit coat over the back of it. "For a Saturday league, some of those guys are out for blood."

"Don't have to tell me twice." Ryan folded his arms and widened his stance. "I wanted to clarify a few things."

Paul sat on the edge of the couch, but didn't say anything.

"If you're truly freaked out by the control issue, then tell me. I need complete honesty from you." Ryan moved to the opposite end of the couch. "You're a natural submissive. You come alive when you give away control. That doesn't happen often. I know what we do might be scary as hell, but it's what we do and it's here. No one else has to see. I don't get into going to the clubs or parading you in public. Why? I don't see the need. That's just me. But I need to know."

Paul stared at his hands before he spoke. He needed to think through how he wanted to answer. "I've never given up control. Usually I'm the one who orchestrates. But maybe that's why my luck with men sucks off the field. I can take orders well, but I never realised it could apply to life." He reached for Ryan. "The parts of our play that scare me aren't because I think you'll hurt me. They scare me because I never thought I'd do any of those things and because I crave them. I crave you. I've never dreamt about anything but art until you came along. I'm willing to do what it takes to make you happy because it's what I need to be happy myself."

"Then you wish to play?" Ryan rubbed the back of Paul's hand with his thumb.

"Oh hells yes." Paul shot out of his seat. "My safe word is cougar and I'm all yours, sir." He offered his wrists. "Play with me?"

"Eager." Ryan rose to his full height. "I've got some new things for you." He grabbed the hem of Paul's shirt and led him to the bedroom. "Undress while I get things ready and don't touch yourself." He kissed Paul on the lips. "I guarantee you'll love this."

When Ryan left the room, Paul couldn't shuck his clothes fast enough. He wadded his jogging pants into a ball then second-guessed himself. What he'd picked up from the bondage porn was that the master expected the sub to be orderly. He shook out his pants then folded them. The pants ended up in a neat pile with the shirt on top and his socks balled. He removed his boxer shorts last, covering the rest of his clothes.

"Very good." Ryan patted Paul's ass. "Tidy. I like it. Now, on your knees."

Paul dropped to the floor, hands behind his back and his head bowed.

"Turn around so I can see you."

When Paul did as Ryan expected, Ryan squatted down before him. "Remember, I want to hear you." He stretched the elastic on a piece of black material. "I'm going to blindfold you. The sensory deprivation will heighten your experience."

"Thank you, sir." A shiver ran up Paul's spine. He closed his eyes as Ryan placed the blindfold over his face. He tried to open them again, but the fabric held his eyes closed. His heart raced and he breathed out through his mouth to calm down.

"Scared?" Ryan touched Paul's chin, his caress light on Paul's skin.

"Excited."

"And so hot." Ryan's breath tickled Paul's cheek. "You turn me on, just looking at you."

Ryan's footsteps padded on the carpet. Paul clasped his fingers together. When the footsteps returned, a clinking sound added to the mix.

"Open." Ryan rubbed something hard against Paul's lips.

Without hesitation, Paul opened his mouth.

"I know I said I wanted you to talk, but I think you'll like this in the short term." He fitted the gag in place in Paul's mouth. "You can still make noise and talk around it. Mostly I want you to get used to the feel." He strapped the ball gag in place. "Feels good, doesn't it?"

Paul nodded. He wanted to say something, but the overwhelming floating feeling came on too strong.

"I'm going to stand you up." Ryan clicked something else and hauled Paul to his feet. Paul knew exactly what Ryan had done. He tried to move his arms. No dice—Ryan had him in the handcuffs. Paul's cock hardened to the point of pain. His balls vibrated and butterflies danced in his chest. Shit, being bound and stripped of his sight did turn him on.

"Jesus, you're hard." Ryan wrapped his hand around Paul's girth and stroked. "It needs something pretty." The footsteps faded then came back louder. "Lots of pretty things for you."

Flat licks and bites peppered Paul's chest. He groaned and fought the bindings. As much as he liked being tied up, he wanted to touch Ryan, to stroke him and show him how much he loved being adored. His body sizzled from his head to his toes.

"Yes, tell me you love this." Ryan pinched Paul's nipple hard, drawing a shimmer of pleasure-filled pain.

Paul groaned and leaned into Ryan. "More, sir," he said around the gag. "Please?"

"I will." Ryan pinched again then left Paul with a burning sensation. "This clip is so sexy against your tanned skin. It glitters."

Paul flexed his hands. The burn on his left nipple abated, only to be replaced by the pinch and delicious pain of the clip on his right nipple.

"This needs a weight." Ryan tugged the chain. "Not much, but enough to let you know it's there." The clamps pulled harder on Paul's nipples and something tapped his belly button. "Lean forward," Ryan commanded.

Although his knees knocked and his legs shook, Paul assumed the position Ryan wanted. The weight skimmed his belly when he moved and the clips bit into his nipples.

"You deserve a treat."

Paul listened for Ryan's next move and his heart skipped a beat when he couldn't hear his lover. Hands splayed on his thighs.

"Can't let this go to waste." Ryan raked his fingernails down Paul's inner thighs and licked the crown of Paul's cock.

"Oh shit," Paul murmured around the gag. He had never expected sex could be so powerful. He groaned and fire licked him from within.

Ryan curled his fingers around Paul's erection then engulfed him in his heat. He flattened his tongue along the underside of Paul's cock then sucked hard. Paul felt the tug from his toes all the way up to his chest.

"Sir. Too close, sir." Paul panted around the ball gag. "Sir."

"You're not thinking of coming, are you?" Ryan clicked something. "I'll have to remedy that." Cool metal surrounded Paul's cock and sac. The cock ring. Blood rushed to his erection and he shook his head. Not being able to see certainly heightened the experience.

"You're being bad, wanting to come already." Ryan abandoned Paul's dick. Clothing rustled and something whooshed past Paul's face. Ryan threaded his fingers into Paul's hair then tilted Paul's head back. "Walk with me."

Paul shuffled his feet and moved where Ryan took him. Giving up control did free him. He didn't have to think, didn't have to worry about anything. With Ryan, the only goal was to enjoy. Ryan eased him forward. Paul bumped something immobile with his knees.

"Just the mattress." Ryan placed his hand on Paul's back. "You're doing so well and so hot, too. Lean over."

Paul did as instructed and waved his ass. "Punish me, sir."

A crack split the air and Paul's ass stung. "Who is in charge here?" Another slap on his butt. "Who?"

"You, sir. Thank you, sir. I deserve another." Paul's words came out garbled around the gag and the sheets.

"Bad boy." Ryan smacked Paul on the ass four more times. "You like your punishment too much."

"Yes, sir." Paul grinned into the mattress. He wanted whatever Ryan could give him. He soared to the highest heights and rode the sexy feelings.

"Mine." Ryan slapped again, but this time Paul lost count of the blows.

The more Ryan spanked him, the more Paul wanted. His cock pulsed between his thigh and the side of the mattress. His nipples ached from the clips and yet, he craved more.

Something behind Paul clicked. Another cock ring? Couldn't be. As far as he knew, Ryan only had the one.

"Mine," Ryan said again. This time he spread Paul's ass cheeks. His breath heated Paul's skin. The scratch of Ryan's day-old whiskers burned on Paul's butt. He fisted his hands and moaned.

Cool liquid dribbled over Paul's hole. Ryan worked one finger into Paul, pushing past the muscle and opening Paul to him. Paul relaxed under Ryan's ministrations. Another spank cracked on his skin. He arched into Ryan's hand.

"So fucking sexy. I'm adding another finger." Ryan speared a second digit into Paul's asshole. The burn faded, replaced by more pleasure.

"I want to hear you." Ryan unbuckled the gag, giving Paul the freedom to speak without garble. "You're doing so well."

"Love it, sir." Paul rode Ryan's fingers. "More, please, sir."

Without saying a word, Ryan added another finger. The pressure mounted in Paul's butt. He'd been filled by the larger butt plug and by Ryan's ass, but three fingers pushed his limits. Ryan curled his index finger and stroked Paul's prostate.

"Fucking God damn," Paul groaned. "More."

"Needy." Ryan added another finger. "You're nearing your limit." He worked his hand in and out of Paul, twisting his fingers and massaging the sweet spot in his ass.

Paul puffed and buried his face in the sheets. "Fuck me, sir. Please. Make me yours." He braced his feet and rolled his hips. Each movement jostled Ryan deep within him.

"Yes." Ryan removed his hand and left Paul bereft.

Paul turned his head. He couldn't see Ryan or hear where he'd gone. Plastic crinkled and something snapped.

"I crave you, too." Ryan grabbed Paul's hips and hoisted him into place. Without giving Paul time to think, Ryan rammed his cock into Paul's ass. Paul gritted his teeth and met Ryan thrust for thrust.

"Do you want to come?" Ryan slapped Paul's butt and surged inside. "Do you?"

"Yes." Paul writhed beneath Ryan. "Need to."

"You can hold it." Ryan smacked again. His rhythm turned jerky and his balls whacked against Paul's. Skin slapped skin and the heady scent of sex and man roved through the room.

"Fuck," Paul bit out. He could hold in the orgasm, but he'd damn well end up exploding.

"Paul." His name came out like a sigh on Ryan's lips. "Oh God."

Ryan's fingers dug into Paul's skin and he pinned Paul to the bed. His cock throbbed within Paul's ass and the extra sensation of coming man turned Paul inside out. Ryan sprawled out on top of him and gasped.

"I didn't forget you, just had to catch my bearings." Ryan kissed Paul's cheek then climbed off him. He pulled out, leaving Paul chilled. "You did very well. So sexy and at my command." Ryan rolled him over and removed the blindfold from Paul's face.

Paul squinted in the bright light. The chain still pulled on his nipples and the handcuffs prevented him from masturbating. He planted his feet and crawled onto the bed. "Felt like heaven."

"Heaven without coming?" Ryan bobbed his eyebrows then stood between Paul's legs. "Come for me. You deserve the release." He curled both hands around Paul's cock and caressed him. The simple, light touches sent Paul's desire spiralling. Paul panted and every muscle in his body went taut. His control snapped.

"Come on me." Ryan aimed Paul's cock in his direction. "Mark me."

"Fuck." Paul succumbed to the orgasm and shot his load all over Ryan's chest. Thick splatters of cum decorated Ryan's pale skin. Ryan dragged his fingers through the mess then leaned over Paul.

"So sexy." He kissed Paul, smearing cum between them.

The handcuffs bit into Paul's back, but he didn't care. The only place he wanted to be was anywhere with Ryan. "You'll need to let me go."

"Not sure I can." Ryan didn't look at Paul. "Let me clean you up." He stood and removed the clips.

Paul sank against the sheets and stared at the ceiling. He had expected something more than just 'not sure I can' from Ryan. Confession of love, maybe?

Ryan returned with a washcloth in hand. "Sit up." Ryan released the handcuffs, then wiped down Paul's chest and covered him with the blanket. "Don't want you to get cold." He left the room again, but came back without the washcloth.

When Ryan settled beside Paul in the bed, Paul found the courage to ask questions. "Is it always going to be like this? You working me into a frenzy but knowing what I can take?" Paul draped his arm across Ryan's chest. "But not giving all of yourself to me?"

"Depends. We can still have quickies and nooners. Those won't go away, but there will always be an element of control in our sex life. You get off on me telling you what to do. I get off on giving you what you need." Ryan held Paul tighter. "Some days we'll have sweet, sensual sex and others will be like today."

"I liked today a lot." Paul nuzzled Ryan's neck. "But we can't dick around for too much longer. I've got a banquet to attend and you're the best arm candy I could ever hope for. "

"You talked me into it." Ryan sat up and scrubbed his hand over his face. "I'll go with you." He glanced over his shoulder. "But we're having a quickie in the shower."

Paul perked up. He had never doubted Ryan, but he loved the way Ryan knew him so well. "Is there any other way to take a shower?"

"Not that I know of." Ryan grinned. "Last one in bottoms." He sprinted naked into the bathroom.

"I am so not losing this bet." Paul chased after Ryan. He wasn't about to let the conversation end—not yet. "One day I hope you'll show me all the black parts of your soul. I'm in love with all of you."

"Just give me time. I will."

Chapter Nine

"This is going to take forever." Paul groaned and toyed with the leftover green beans on his plate. He hadn't been able to eat since he and Ryan had sat down for dinner. His mind was jumbled with memories of their time together and the thing Ryan had said. Forever couldn't come fast enough. Paul leaned in close to Ryan. "I want to go home and do all the things we did all over again."

"Me too. But you've got to accept your award." Ryan shifted in his seat and patted Paul's thigh. "Even if you weren't supposed to know about it. You've practised a speech, haven't you?"

"No, I plan on getting up there and making an ass of myself." Paul shredded his napkin. The one thing he hadn't come clean to Ryan about weighed on his mind. "I've got a surprise for you at the house. I meant to show you and never got a chance." Bullshit he had never got the chance. He snorted. Compared to Ryan's artwork, what he had completed looked amateurish.

"Oh?" Ryan speared the last couple of green beans with his fork. "A surprise, huh?" He nodded as he finished his dinner. "Cool."

"We're here tonight to recognise the Teacher of the Year. Normally our very own Paul Toth does the winner's painting. This year we thought we'd shake things up a bit. On the recommendation of my friend Professor Dolton Pride, we found our artist. I'd like to recognise the artist for this year's portrait...Ryan Malone." George Laubenthal clapped his hands. His glasses slid down his nose. "Stand up so we can recognise you. Ladies and gentlemen, you probably know him more than you think."

Albeit slowly, Ryan stood and waved. A deep blush swept across his cheeks, down his chin and ended somewhere below his collar. The hand he kept at his side balled into a fist. Paul straightened out Ryan's fingers and rubbed his thumb across the back of Ryan's hand. He wanted to say something to release the tension, but until Laubenthal had finished the speech, Ryan wouldn't calm down.

"Oh, you don't have to hide, Mr Malone. We're all big fans." George clapped again. "Your collection at the museum is some of the best art I've ever seen."

"It is," Paul murmured. "I'm your biggest fan."

Ryan blew out a long breath, sat down then massaged the bridge of his nose. "This is your night, not mine."

"It's ours." Paul wrapped an arm around Ryan. "Wouldn't have it any other way. And besides, he didn't mention what you want to forget, so it's all good."

"True." Ryan relaxed a bit and opened the top button on his suit coat.

"And now," George Laubenthal interjected, "our Teacher of the Year this year has been with us for quite a long time. Eight years of service, dedicated to the education of our students. While I can't tell you the difference between a Monet and a Manet, he can. The new curriculum for the freshman programme integrating art into each subject for enrichment is working out well. The students benefit from the extra time and effort spent in ensuring their education is the best."

"He's babbling." Paul shook his head. He'd done plenty for the school district, but to be singled out…he wasn't so sure he wanted the award any longer.

"Enjoy the limelight," Ryan whispered. "It doesn't last forever."

"For outstanding service, above and beyond the educational standards," Laubenthal continued, "we recognise Paul Toth. Congratulations, Mr Toth."

Ryan's words stuck with Paul. The limelight might not last forever, but who wanted forever without love? He grinned. He'd found his forever with Ryan. Paul rose from his seat and strode to the podium. With Laubenthal's help, he grabbed the corner of the sheet covering the painting. Normally, he stood at the back of the room happily cheering on whoever won. The unveiling wasn't difficult, but the anticipation would kill him. The sheet slid off the painting and the breath wrenched from Paul's chest.

The oil painting reminded him of a photograph. Very few visible brushstrokes and perfect attention to fine detail. He trailed his fingers over the heavy oak frame. Damn. The gallery works were nothing compared to the portrait. Paul glanced back at Ryan. The first moment he could corner Ryan he'd ask why Ryan had ever bothered to play football when his natural artistic talents trumped any kicking skills.

"You know we want to hear a speech." Laubenthal grinned and stepped away from the podium.

Paul touched the frame once more then took his place at the mic. "There are a lot of things I could say right now that would be really boring. I could talk about how I wanted to be a teacher from the moment I went to kindergarten. Or explain how I came up with the cross-curricular curriculum. But I can't. Thank you to all those who deemed me worthy of this honour. I'm thrilled beyond comprehension. Thank you. But winning this award also showed me that being the best doesn't always mean you can't learn. I thought I knew a lot about art and life. Turns out what I knew didn't amount to much. It took crossing the line and putting my heart out where it could be stomped on to make me see what really mattered. So once again, thank you. I'm honoured you've chosen me, but moreover, thank you, Ryan. Without you, I'm sure I'd never be the same."

Ryan sank back in his seat. The one thing he had never expected Paul to say out loud, he'd said. He'd outed the both of them. Somehow, he wasn't upset. He liked knowing the world knew about them.

Paul dipped his head and strode from the stage. He shook hands with each of the board members and snagged hugs from quite a few of the faculty. When he returned to the table, his tie hung crooked and his shirt was wrinkled in a couple of spots.

"You look like you ran a gauntlet." Ryan adjusted Paul's tie. "Did they leave me anything?"

Paul sat down in unison with Ryan. "I meant every word up there."

"I know." Ryan rested his arm on the back of his seat and turned to fully face Paul. Time to unburden himself and to admit what he'd known all along. "When I started playing ball, I did it for something to do. I never planned on 'going pro'. The coaches wanted that career path for me. I spent my free time in the museums and in the galleries on campus. I wanted to paint for a living. When the NFL called and told me I was up for the draft, I blew it off. No one drafts a kicker. But they did and I ended up with the Bengals. I loved the game and my team, so it never occurred to me I'd chosen the wrong path in life."

"It wasn't wrong, just winding." Paul inched closer to Ryan. "Got you here, didn't it?"

"You're right. I thought I knew what I wanted from life, until Duke fucked me over. I shut down and kept my nose to the ground. No one saw me and no one hurt me." Ryan held Paul's hand. His limbs trembled and his tongue felt sixteen sizes too big for his mouth, but he pushed forward. "Then you showed up. You turned everything upside down when you walked into that locker room. My heart started. It'd never really stopped, but I felt like I'd started over. Crazy, huh?"

"Not crazy at all." Paul smoothed his thumb across Ryan's chin. "I'm happy to belong to you. Happiest I've ever been and unless you toss my ass out, I'm yours. Forever."

Now for the hard part. Ryan gathered his courage and stared into Paul's eyes. "I love you, Paul." He held his breath, awaiting Paul's answer.

"Yeah?" Paul wrapped his arm around Ryan. "I love you, too."

Ryan stared at Paul for what seemed like an eternity. "I love hearing you say that."

"Love you so much," Paul said. He kissed Ryan on the lips. "So much."

Ryan rested his forehead against Paul's. Relief swept through Ryan and he cupped Paul's jaw in his hand.

A shadow stepped between them and the light. "Get a room." George Laubenthal laughed and held his belly. "I guess he wasn't so shy after all, was he, Paul?"

Paul's eyes widened and his mouth opened a fraction of an inch.

"Thank you, Ryan, for the painting. We'll be in touch next year. I'd also like to talk to you later about acquiring some of your work for the school." George offered his hand. "Paul knows where to find me. And, Paul, congratulations." He shook hands with both Ryan and Paul then strolled off.

"He never ceases to amaze me." Ryan tapped his fingers over his mouth. "The guy seems so proper until you talk to him. Then he's like a goofy old man."

"And he says the damnedest things. He told me you were shy and not what I expected. Guess he was right all along—even if you're not shy." Paul turned his attention back to Ryan. "The party lasts for another hour, but there's something else I want to do tonight and it's not partying with the faculty."

"Mr Toth, are you asking me to take you home?" Ryan feigned horror then chuckled. He lowered his voice to a whisper and spoke in Paul's ear. "Or are you trying to convince me to whisk you out of here for a celebratory spanking? I bought a brand new flogger with your name on it. Goes along with the black rope we used earlier." An image of the toy came to mind. Black glass handle with thick strips of leather dangling from one end.

"Oh God." Paul shivered.

"Multi-purpose," Ryan whispered. His tongue grazed Paul's earlobe when he enunciated the 'l' in multi. "Multiple ways to satisfy you."

"This is so not the time to discuss this," Paul groaned. Hunger burned bright in his eyes and he opened and closed his mouth like he wanted to say something.

"I've rendered you speechless?" Ryan trailed his fingers over Paul's cheek. "You are so sexy when you're stunned. Makes me want to take you home and strap you down to my bed so I can take advantage of you."

Paul grabbed Ryan's arm. "Someone could hear us and that's part of what's turning me on." He rested his forehead on Ryan's. "The rest is all you. I'm nothing, especially not the man who wins awards, without you. Think we can grab the painting and slip out without anyone noticing?"

"We crossed the lines before with fantastic results," Ryan replied. "You take care of the painting and I'll bring the Jeep around."

"Then you'll punish me for being a bad boy?" Paul wiggled his eyebrows. "All night long with that flogger and the clips? I've been pretty damned naughty."

Ryan tossed his head back and laughed. He couldn't have found a more perfectly flawed man if he had tried and he didn't want to. He loved Paul Toth with his entire heart. "I'll please you all night long with whatever you want. I'm yours, too."

"Hot damn. Let's go home."

IN THE RED ZONE

Stephanie Burke

Dedication

This book goes out to Wendi Zwaduk and Cheryl Dragon, who threw a Hump Day Hump dare back at me. It is for my Facebook friends who encouraged it, my family who endured me writing it, and to my Beta Reader Mona who laughed at me for getting trapped in my own challenge before yelling at me to write faster. Mostly, this is for my son who still won't look at hot guys with me because he identifies as intelligence-sexual and not crazy enough to go there with his mother...I love my brat.

Chapter One

"Twenty-seven! Thirty-six! Fifteen—hike!"

In the back of his mind, Dolton heard the words. His blood jumped at the sound of the snap, but his eyes were focused in on his goal.

The quarterback from his rival team, the Rockville Rocs, was going down.

He watched as the quarterback stepped back, looking for a receiver, and Dolton thought to himself, *Not today*.

He dodged to his left, avoiding the defensive lineman who was attempting to keep the pocket, the grouping of men using their bodies as a wall to protect the quarterback, and neatly slipped in between two of them. He caught a glimpse of movement off to his right, but instead of slowing down, he hunkered lower and kept moving, ploughing everything out of his path. Dolton was not the tallest man on the team but he made his low centre of gravity and his ability to slide through tight spots work for him.

The quarterback never saw what hit him.

"That is a sack, folks, and the end of this game! The play clock has run out and the Griffins have tossed back the Rocs like so much cheap beer!"

Dolton didn't pay much attention to the announcers or the quarterback who was crushed beneath his weight. His new focus was on a glorious head of blond hair trailing down the back of a gold and black jersey.

Dean Majors, right tackle, all-around good guy and of late, the star of his masturbation fantasies, placed his hands on the ground, his head low and his ass high in the air before he gave up and rolled himself onto his back. Huffing in exhaustion, he extended his right hand up towards Dolton for assistance.

Feeling his heartbeat beginning to race, Dolton reached for the hand, gripping it tightly just as the rest of the team enveloped them, tossing Dolton in the air and yanking his hands from Dean's grasp.

The disconnection was almost painful.

"Dolton! Dol-ton! Dol-ton!" His name was being chanted as he was carried triumphantly off the field, but Dolton couldn't resist turning back one more time to stare at the mass of blond hair now revealed fully as Dean pulled off his helmet.

Sparkling blue eyes met his and for a moment, Dolton felt like he had been punched in the chest. But that feeling passed quickly as a brown-haired man enveloped him in a massive hug, lifting him off his feet and spinning him around.

Dolton lost sight of Dean and Robbie as the team carried him into the locker rooms and to the grinning face of their manager Tina Edmonson.

"I am so proud of you," the portly Asian woman chuckled. "So very proud. The Rocs are no pushovers, but you guys handed them their collective asses!"

She paused as more cheering echoed around the state-of-the-art locker room. Dolton was grateful that his university had such a modern place for them to practise and recover. Of course the local weekend league only used the field when the college team wasn't bent on killing each other to impress the scouts during the season, but it was a privilege for them to be able to use the same equipment and facilities.

"And because you guys did so well, next game we face our rivals the Dragons."

There was good-natured booing and hissing which was more amusing than threatening. If anybody sounded like a bunch of overgrown lizards at the moment, it had to be them.

"So rest up and avail yourselves of the Jacuzzi and steam room if need be, and I will see you all next week to go over strategy and look at film."

There was one final cheer for their totally badass performance on the field then Tina was slipping out so they could get on with the business of getting clean and comfortable.

And for Dolton that meant looking for Dean and getting as close to him as he could in the showers to get more fodder for his spank bank.

Yes, he was a healthy twenty-nine-year-old and masturbated frequently. He was never ashamed of that particular bodily function and loved to share in the joys of self-love with whomever he was seeing at the time, though right now he wasn't seeing anyone.

He desired to change that real soon, he reminded himself, as he moved towards his locker and his waiting toiletry kit.

Some of the guys on the small seventeen-man team had slipped out, preferring to get cleaned up at home, and Dolton silently prayed that this was one of those times when most of the guys rolled out and left him and Dean alone in the lockers.

Oh yeah, that was a fantasy he didn't want to examine too closely — him tying Dean to the inclined bench in the weight room, gagging him with his sweaty jock, and fucking the hell out of the blond. He would squirm so deliciously under him, he decided, and was really beginning to lose himself in his musings when a sharp slap brought him back to the present.

"Reliving those glory moments?" a boisterous voice asked and internally Dolton winched as Robbie Keton invaded his personal body space. Had the man ever heard of boundaries?

"Something like that," he answered, his growing erection wilting at the sound of the man. He turned to look at him, noting that Robbie had already stripped off his jersey and his shoulder pads.

"You did great out there, thought if you want some tips to improve your game —"

"Lay off our middle linebacker," a quiet man named Aiden growled, stepping to Dolton's side and handing him a bottle of cold water. To prevent himself from having to say anything, Dolton twisted off the cap and downed half the bottle on one gulp.

"Just helping out, Aiden," Robbie conceded, lifting his hands in a surrendering motion. "Don't need to get all defensive. I was a pro, you know. And I just wanted to point out some weak spots that I saw."

"When we want your professional opinion, we'll beat it out of you, okay, Keton?" Aiden snapped, totally dismissing the guy and turning back to Dolton. "You did good out there, little man."

"Little." Dolton snorted, flexing the arm not holding onto the bottle. "Not in your lifetime, old man."

Dolton looked over at Robbie, noted the frown on his face before the man turned to harass Dean some more.

"I don't know why we let that guy play," Aiden muttered, also watching the irritant's retreat. "There are so many good players out there we could have that come with the off switch that dude seems to lack."

"He was NFL," Dolton pointed out.

"National Fucking Lunatics, yeah, I can see that."

Dolton's snort of laughter drew attention to them as more of the players came over to congratulate him on his awesome hit.

In the ensuing chaos, he lost sight of Dean and Robbie. Sucking his teeth in disappointment, he stripped off his jersey and protective gear and made his way to the showers.

There were only a few guys taking advantage and because none of them were Dean, he had no trouble keeping his erection down. When he was done, he didn't sit in the whirlpool tub, but instead dressed swiftly and headed for home.

Next week he would ensure that he spent some time talking to the delicious Dean and maybe even convince him to go out for coffee or something.

Next week, he decided, he would definitely make his move — as soon as he came up with a plan.

* * * *

Dean winced, rubbing his left shoulder as a deep ache began to set in. He knew it would take some time in the Jacuzzi at home to ease the ache, but the small pain was worth it.

He had seen the huge blocker from the Rocs get a lock on Dolton and had almost flipped his shit. There was no way he was going to let that beautiful black man get bruises all over that toffee-coloured skin.

His body had reacted before his mind had caught up and he had found himself hitting the guy low in the gut, flattening him and leaving Dolton free to take the tackle.

He had hopped to his feet as soon as the play was dead and reached for Dolton, who had looked up at him from between the guards of his helmet, and Dean could have sworn he had read something in his eyes before the rest of the team had carried him away.

He had watched the man he wanted to bang like the fists of an angry god get away. His only consolation prize was Robbie racing over to hug the shit out of him.

Even in the locker room there was always someone slapping him on the shoulder, talking about the awesome block he had made or Robbie running off at the mouth.

Dean just smiled and nodded to most of the bullshit his old friend was spouting, finding it easier to just ignore the hell out of Robbie most times, but he was starting to get really irritating. He watched as the loud-spoken man waded thought the clash of players to talk to Dolton, who suddenly developed a long-suffering look on his face. He was about to intervene when Aiden interrupted and Robbie walked off in a huff.

"All I wanted to do was give him some advice," Robbie was droning on as he complained to him about how stuck-up some of the players were. "And he just dismissed me. Me, Dean? I was All Star for the Cornhuskers and then first-round draft for the Cowboys. My advice is golden."

And your busted knee that got you off the team was almost a bigger disaster then your mouth – which was going to get you off the team anyway, Dean thought, but merely rolled his eyes at his old friend. It was amazing how a few years and a wad of cash could change someone.

Robbie used to be one of the most open-minded people he knew. They had met in high school and had become fast friends, only losing touch when Robbie went off to university and he went off to a trade school. They had kept in touch periodically before the draft and Robbie's meteoric rise to fame. That was the last he'd heard from his old friend until a surprise call from the man himself netted him the story of Robbie's busted knee and how it had landed him right back in their hometown once more.

It had been Dean's suggestion that Robbie joined their weekend league, some time for them to reacquaint and use his pro ball knowledge to better the team, a suggestion that he was now regretting with every fibre of his being.

Robbie had dramatically changed while he'd been away, turning into the world's biggest asshole. Of course Robbie had been a bit of a jerk in high school, but he'd never gone in for picking on the kids that were in lower grades or considered geeks by his jock friends. He had been a little above everyone who was not on the team…and Dean, but he never set out make himself better than anyone else. But now he was rapidly surpassing 'asshole' and speeding straight towards 'cunt'-dom.

"You would think —"

"Give it a rest, yeah?" Dean finally asked, exasperated beyond belief. "Sure, we all can use your advice," Dean placated as he began pulling off his gear. "But wait until someone asks for it, okay, man? This is not the NFL, Robbie. Most of these guys are playing for fun or to get out of the house for a few hours." Dean cut him off, not in the mood for any more of his attitude. "So give it a rest until next week. And my shoulder is throbbing."

"That boy should have taken better care to plan his attack and maybe you would've not been hurt."

"What the fuck?" Not believing what his friend had just said, Dean slowly turned around, his shoulder pads in hand, and glared at his friend.

"He is younger than the rest of us," Robbie was quick to explain. "I didn't mean anything by it, man. You know that. I'm not that person."

"That *boy*," Dean emphasised the word, "is an adjunct professor of literature, Robbie. Not just English lit, literature — which means he speaks and reads about five different languages. He has spent time in some of the most remote, Godforsaken areas in the world to advance his learning and did it all before he turned thirty. He may be younger, but there is nothing 'boy' about him, in any sense of the word."

"What are you, his fan club?" Robbie blushed a little, obviously set aback by Dean's defence of Dolton. "If you like him so much, why don't you marry him?"

"I wish," Dean mumbled under his breath before shaking his head at his old friend. "Just watch what you say and how you say it. Most of these guys would pound your face into the concrete before you got to try and explain yourself."

"So they are sensitive little babies," Robbie teased. "I'll try and not hurt their feelings."

"Fuck you, Robbie," Dean snorted, storing his pads and jerseys in a huge carry-all before toeing off his cleats and tossing them inside. He slipped on a pair of shower shoes and slammed his locker shut.

"Fuck you too, Majors," Robbie laughed back, slapping him on the sore shoulder. "You taking off?"

"Yeah," Dean grudgingly admitted, shrugging his shoulder to relieve some of the stiffness as he felt a headache brewing under his temples. "I'll clean up at home."

"We should get together—"

"Not today, Robbie," Dean sighed. "My shoulder is busted and my head is pounding, I just want to get clean and catch a nap."

"I understand, man." Robbie nodded before turning to make his way to his own locker. "I'll see you soon."

"Not if I can help it," he muttered under his breath, turning to look for Dolton again and not finding him through the crush of people near his locker.

Maybe that was for the best, he decided. There was no way he could hide the boner he knew he was going to throw at the sight of Dolton's dark skin and sexy bald head. Not that anyone would have cared, but horny shower room stalker was not the image he wanted to maintain.

Dean was as queer as a three-dollar bill and was not ashamed of it. You would not find him marching in any parades or hoisting flags at rallies, but he was open and honest to all those who cared to ask—his family and his close friends and of course his business partner. After all, his business partner had been the one to give Dean his first blow job and lead him into the temptation that was an anal orgasm. Ever since then, he had not even tried to deny his orientation to himself, let alone anyone else who cared to know. But now there was only one person he was interested in knowing all about his majorly hot deep-throating skills, and that was Dolton.

He was sure that he had a shot, catching the educated younger man staring at him a few times with lust in his eyes, but neither had yet made a move. And with Robbie's ignorance still stewing in his head, he thought it best to put some space between him and his old friend even if it meant leaving the presence of his fantasy love god.

Besides, he was quite sure he was going to have to knock Robbie the fuck out the moment Robbie found out he was gay and his shoulder was aching too much for that fight.

He tiredly clomped out of the locker room with a few of the team who were also travelling home to clean up, and stomped over to his extra duty pickup truck.

Sure, it was a manly-man penis extension, but he really needed it for work. Sometimes even the boss had to go to the construction site and get his hands dirty. And as the best electrician in the Tri-State area, he found himself often visiting several work sites in a day and troubleshooting everything from damaged cables to wiring stereo equipment. His truck had to be large enough to carry a variety of equipment — plus the jacked-up pickup looked cool as fuck.

He often fantasised about fucking the hell out of Dolton in the crew cab.

Chuckling at his own depravity, Dean started the engine and made his way home for a hot bath, a quick bite, and a huge jack-off session with his favourite dildo. If images of Dolton spread out on his bed begging for it appeared in his horny mind, it would make his evening better. All in all, it was not such a bad way to spend a Sunday afternoon.

Chapter Two

"Man do I have problems." The swirling water around Dolton's body was not helping matters any. He looked down balefully at the book in his hands and decided that even eighteenth-century Japanese erotic love poetry was not going to take his mind off his issues.

Dean Majors. There was something about the man that made him want to push him ass up over the nearest surface and eat the fuck out of his ass. Of course that would lead to him fucking him through whatever surface they were utilising —

The surge in his cock made him place his book on the floor outside the tub and stare at his swollen length.

As easy as it would be to just grip it and take care of business on his own, he was hungry for more. He wanted Dean on his knees with his lips wrapped around the thick base. He wanted Dean on his back with his legs spread open, his hungry hole winking at him. He wanted Dean on his knees offering his ass up for the taking while he fisted his cock in his eagerness.

There were so many things he wanted but for once in his life he was unsure how to proceed.

Dean was definitely not a woman in need of being wooed and he was sure that the man would not appreciate any attempts at romance with candy and flowers. That wasn't his style and he was sure that Dean would probably curse him out faster than kiss him if he took that route.

He could go for the aggressive play and just slam the man against the locker room wall and have at it, but Dean's friendship with Robbie Keton made him hesitate in approaching him out of anything but friendship. Robbie was an asshole but Dean had never behaved in that manner. It was food for thought.

But that was doing nothing to help his little problem.

Dolton looked over his body, past the colourful tattoos that covered large portions of him and at the thick swelling at his groin. His dick seemed to have developed a mind of its own now and it wanted Dean with a passion.

There was no help for it. Lathering up his hand, he rose to his knees so that his cock just barely kissed the water.

He gripped his wayward dick in one hand, cupping his balls in the other and began to work them.

He moaned, closing his eyes and he let his head fall back as the image of Dean and that perfect bubble butt of his came into his mind's eye.

God, the blond was hot. He was a little taller than Dolton but his body was firm and muscular. And his hair…it framed a face that had the most beautiful plump red lips and a pair of arresting aqua blue eyes. It flowed down his back like liquid gold.

Dolton's fist pumped faster as shards of pleasure began racing along his spine.

Dean's voice was a deep drawl—the kind of voice that would only get rough and gravelly when he grew aroused—and he could hear him calling his name.

He wanted to bend that man over and spread him open and just dive in. His flesh would be succulent and pink and Dolton was sure that he was the type to let out tight little whimpers while he ate his ass. Oh yeah, he was going to bury his face between his cheeks and feast like a starving man.

Dean would wiggle and press his ass back further into his mouth—he would spread his own cheeks wide and demand that Dolton treat his hole right.

He began to pull at the head of his dick faster and tug at his balls as his dream Dean rolled onto his knees and wiggled his ass at him.

"Come and get it, baby," he would demand, his hair flowing beautiful and bright over his body as he stared at him over his shoulder. *"Come on, fuck my ass and blow your load inside."*

Dean would be soft like cotton inside, hot and slick and soft and wrapped tightly around him.

"Damn, baby," Dean would moan as Dolton slid into him. Dolton was not a small man in the dick department and he could picture Dean's eyes growing wider and wider as he was split, drilled and filled with each thick inch.

Dolton was groaning now, the sound of his own lust adding to his pleasure as he gave himself over fully to the fantasy.

Dean would buck and scream under him, his hole sucking him in deep as his fingers sank into his back, demanding he be taken harder, faster, stronger.

Dean's cock would be pink, the head as scarlet as his lips as he gave himself fully to his fucking, pushing his ass higher and begging for it, begging him for dick.

Dolton's hand was a blur as he squeezed himself almost painfully tight. That was how tight Dean's lily-white ass would be.

And he would force his way into that tight hole and paint his insides with his cum, marking him so that no one would ever look at him with lust again.

Dean was his and he was going to fuck him and pull out and blow his load all over his face, those pretty red lips, that perfect ass —

"Dean!" he shouted as his balls slammed up, as lightning ran through his body and his cock began to shoot. "Fuck!" he gasped, sinking back into the hot water for a moment to calm his breathing. All too soon he had to get out, drain the tub and shower the remains of his flights into fantasy away.

His dream Dean was purring though, his face covered in his jizz as he lapped the creamy cum from his lips.

It was a picture that carried him into peaceful dreams that night and would fuel his imagination until he could get the real thing into his bed — where he belonged.

Chapter Three

"Good practice."

Dolton looked up from his book to glare at his friend Ryan Malone as he plopped down on the bench beside him. He closed his book and stared out over the playing field. The rest of his team were packing it in, moving towards the locker rooms while those who watched from the stands were quietly leaving the stadium.

Their practice had been rudimentary, just a going over of plays before they faced their rivals the Dragons. Having the Dragons' former star kicker suddenly appear out of the blue was just an occupational hazard as he was doing a job at the university.

"Stealing plays for your girlfriends?" he joked, watching the man snort in laughter.

"Like we need help to grind your stupid asses into the dirt."

"Fuck you, Malone." Dolton chuckled, placing his book aside to look his friend and sometime associate over. Ryan was an artist and often seemed like the only one in this whole town who had common sense. "What are you doing here anyway?"

"Was passing by when I saw you reading Taketori Monogatari and figured if you were reading something as depressing as seventh-century Japanese science fiction bamboo girls abandoning their families for the greater good, then you are having personal problems."

"I need to get laid."

"And on that note, hope you have a good day."

Ryan made to stand up when Dolton threw his book at him. His friend deftly caught the ancient tome and solemnly handed it back. "You done acting like a six-year-old girl?"

"Fuck you."

"No, I am not on your getting laid agenda. So are you going to tell me what's bothering you or are you going to throw another temper tantrum?"

Dolton looked out over the field where special teams were running plays then turned his attention to his left where Dean was patiently listening to that ass Robbie Keton expound on something with a lot of flailing arms and aggressive gestures.

"God, no," Ryan moaned, shaking his head as he turned to follow Dolton's gaze to the pair. "Please tell me you are not into rough trade with assholes."

"Robbie?" Dolton felt his face wrinkle in disgust as he glared at his friend. "Not even if his was the last hole open for business on the face of the earth."

"Then it must be the pretty blond."

"Dean Majors, a hot man, a stunning personality, and the ass of death." He tilted his head as Dean rolled his eyes at his companion and squatted with one knee on the ground, effectively pointing that perfect ass in their direction while he rested.

"Yeah." Ryan tilted his head to the side. "I see what you mean."

"Practically perfect in every way." Dolton turned away from the object of his desire and looked to his friend once more. "And friends with a retard. See my dilemma?"

"No. You want to fuck Blondie, not his redneck friend."

"Before, I was sure I had a shot. Now that he brought Asshole into the picture, I am not so sure."

"So ask him."

"Just walk over and ask him if he would like to bend over and let me partake of his fine ass?"

"Why not?" Ryan rose to his feet, his chest heaving as he silently laughed at his friend. "Worst he can say is no. And from the way he keeps stealing looks at you, I am quite sure your blue balls problem will be a thing of the past." Dolton glared, but Ryan just laughed. "Thanks for the recommendation. I got the job painting that mural."

"You can be an ass, but at least you are a talented one. The work you reproducing those woodcuts found in those ancient Japanese wall panels is still being talked about over at the museum."

"Talking," Ryan nodded. "A novel approach to solving a problem. Maybe it should be something you look into. I hear it works wonders." Ryan smirked outright as he walked away, leaving Dolton glaring at his retreating back.

"Bastard," Dolton grumbled under his breath, but then their coach was calling for the defensive line-up and he placed his book back on the bench and moved to join his team on the field.

Out of curiosity, he looked in Dean's direction and realised Ryan was right as Dean quickly glanced away, pulling his flowing hair back into a tail before he smushed his helmet over his head. Maybe he had a shot after all.

But as his quarterback began to call plays, he put his mind back into the game. Suddenly his path was clear. He knew what he was going to do. Tonight, Dean Majors would be in his bed or he would set his sights on more willing prey.

* * * *

Dean was staring and the stupid thing was that he knew he was going to get caught. Fact of the matter was that he really didn't care.

Dolton was looking exceptionally fine, his muscles pumped to the fullest and he was doing that intelligence thing, reading away at a book that Dean would probably find incomprehensible. Not that he was lacking in intelligence but few people's brains operated on the level that Dolton's did so easily.

He felt his heart stop when a very handsome dark-haired man walked over and easily started a conversation with him. For a moment he was sure that the man he wanted was taken, but they didn't treat each other like lovers. His relief was so great that he had to squat down or he was going to fall on his ass. It got a puzzled reaction from Robbie, but he did as he usually did and ignored his childhood friend and kept stealing glances at Dolton.

All too soon the defensive line was being called to the field to run plays and Dean found himself too busy to think about anything but the plays being called.

But now, after practice, when they were all filing in or clearing out of the locker room, Dolton was still sitting and reading that small book.

"My house? Brews?" Robbie asked and Dean made some excuse as he moved towards his target.

"But we never spend any time together," Robbie was complaining. "And the way you're staring at Baldie over there makes me think you got a crush on him or something."

"Jesus, Robbie," Dean hissed, flushing because Robbie was not one for keeping his voice low. He looked around to see if Dolton had heard and groaned softly as he saw those golden-brown eyes boring straight into his. He turned away to glare at his friend. "You just don't know what to say out of your fucking mouth."

"Well, it's not like you are making it easy to hang with you, man. I've been here months and I can never catch up with you."

"It takes a lot to run a business, Robbie," Dean offered, and it was the truth...mostly. "I don't get a lot of time to myself." He was beginning to look distressed, he knew, and was moments from telling him he thought Robbie had turned into an egotistical prick that he didn't want to waste his time with. He had spent an evening with Robbie once, and after a night of beer-swilling and loud trash-talking, he had decided it was an event he didn't care to repeat. Before he could say anything else to dissuade Robbie, Dolton rose to his feet and walked over to them.

"So, Dean, you ready to discuss my electrical problem?"

The man was hot and sweaty, still wearing his practice pants and a T-shirt, though he had removed and stored his pads. His eyes — they were amused and hungry. Dean fought the urge to demand he be fucked right now and turned to Robbie.

"Like I said, man, business calls. Not all of us have a NFL salary to draw from."

"Yeah." Robbie looked from him to Dolton and back again before he nodded slowly. "Yeah. Lucky me." He flashed his trademark grin and slapped Dean on the shoulder. He shot Dolton a derisive glare before he turned and made his way towards the showers.

"Charming friend you got there." Dolton shook his head, tapping the book he still carried against one bulging thigh.

"Isn't he just." Dean shook his head, refusing to apologise for the man. Robbie was a big boy. If he had to suck up to anyone at a later date he could do that on his own. "Thank you for that. You really didn't have to."

"Oh yes, I did." Dolton smiled, his white teeth glinting like a model in a toothpaste ad. "I really need to talk to you."

Dean looked back towards the showers, where Robbie was no doubt irritating the masses with his own brand of humour, and to the hot guy he wanted to fuck. *Hot guy wins every time.* "Here or..."

"My place," Dolton decided and Dean nodded in acceptance. "There is something there I need to show you."

"Shower?" he asked and bit back a moan as Dolton smirked at him.

"You can use the one I have at my place. It's not too far from campus. I like to live near where I work."

"Then I'm all yours."

The answering grin he got in return made his dick swell and his imagination race.

He looked over Dolton, the colourful tats on his built body, the intelligent wickedness behind his eyes, those full lips that would look mighty fine wrapped around his cock...if that man but asked, he really would be all his. He would make damn sure of it.

Chapter Four

"Beautiful place," Dean murmured as they walked into his house.

"Thank you." Dolton smiled as they entered his two-storey abode about a mile away from the campus. "It's a place I can hang my hat."

They stepped across the stone hallway and into the sunken living room where Dean's mouth dropped open. Dolton was proud of his home and he had filled it with the treasures he had discovered as he travelled the world. He loved Dean's reaction to the things he held most dear.

He watched as Dean stepped down the five stairs and walked across the marble floor towards a display case that held his precious artefacts from Japan.

"One of my favourite places to travel is Asia, Japan in particular."

"You are an anthropologist, I understand," Dean murmured before his eyes strayed to a mounted katana, the katana, the wakizashi, and the tanto's sheaths covered in the most beautiful red leather Dolton himself had ever seen.

"Among other things," Dolton answered, taking in his prey. Dean was wearing a loose pair of track pants that beautifully caressed that perfect bubble butt he loved to flaunt. His muscular upper body was covered in a baggy white T-shirt that was so old and thin he might as well be naked. On his feet was a pair of black slides he wore in place of his cleats. His sports bag was slung over his shoulder and his hair was pulled back into a messy tail at the base of his neck and trailed over his shoulder in dark blond waves.

He was so asking to get fucked.

"You wanted my opinion, Pride?" he asked, his bright blue eyes darkening to almost navy as they trailed over his body. "From what I can see, you don't need electric help."

Oh yeah, this boy was down.

"Yeah." Dolton gathered his courage and stepped over into Dean's personal space. "I need help" — he leant down and smirked as Dean sucked in a deep breath, his pupils dilating — "in the attic."

He spun on his heel and began to walk away, expecting Dean to follow. A quick peek over his shoulder showed that Dean was, his eyes travelling over his décor that ran from strange to outright exotic.

"You've been all over the world," he commented softly as they made their way to the spiral staircase that led to the upper floors.

"Pretty much." Dolton paused to look over his shoulder, noting that Dean jerked his eyes up from where they had been examining his ass. "And I always bring back souvenirs."

He watched as Dean blushed and swore he would be balls deep in the quiet man soon.

"The attic is through the bedroom," he added and adjusted himself where Dean could get an eyeful of what he was packing.

The other man swallowed hard and nodded, his own pants beginning to tent.

True to his word, Dolton led the blond through his bedroom, grinning when Dean paused at the huge California king-sized bed draped in while silk and the matching fluttering curtains at the huge sliding glass doors that led to a deck.

"Through here." Dolton drew his attention to a large doorway that held another set of wide spiralling stairs.

The attic was a huge room with vaulted ceilings and a glowing redwood floor. In the centre of the room was a large circular bed covered in white fur. There were two large windows tinted in dark glass that allowed in the sunlight but prevented anyone from the outside looking in. There was a huge circular chandelier hanging over the bed and bookcases framed in recessed lighting lined the walls.

"You want to add more light?" Dean asked, unable to tear his eyes away from the fur-covered bed. "This den is perfect."

"It's more of a play room..." Dolton trailed off as Dean jerked his eyes up to his.

"You didn't bring me here for my opinion, did you?" Dean's voice dropped an octave when he grew aroused.

"Oh, I do need your opinion." Swift as a hunting cat, Dolton made his move. Before the other man could blink, he was in his face, one hand going to his hair tie to free his hair, the other gripping his chin and forcing him to look down at him. Dean was maybe an inch taller than him, but that wouldn't matter when he was flat on his back with his legs in the air. "When I fuck you, do you want to be on your knees or on your back? Think carefully 'cause that is the only decision you get."

"I don't have a choice?" Dean arched his eyebrow at him and Dolton felt his erection jump in his pants.

"You knew what you were getting into when you walked into my house."

"True."

Dolton liked that—honesty was important to him. He reached out and pulled Dean's bag from his shoulder and dropped it to the floor. "There is a shower in the corner." He leaned in and lapped at Dean's lips, feeling his lust rise as Dean closed his eyes and relaxed into him. "We are going over there and I am going to peel you and wash you. Then I am laying you face first on that fur and eating your ass until you beg me to fuck you."

Dean practically pulled him to the shower.

The small bathroom was more serviceable than anything else, a white glass shower stall large enough for two, a sink and a toilet.

Once inside the door, Dean threw his arms around Dolton and began to devour his mouth. Dolton relaxed and let him, pushing back with his tongue and taking over the kiss after a moment. Dean moaned into his mouth, so delicious, but Dolton pulled away.

"Before this goes any further, there are some things you need to know about me." He looked down at Dean, at his passion-swollen lips, his glittering eyes, his heaving chest, and had to take a step back before he just jumped him—to hell with proprieties.

"Things?" Dean panted, his eyes intent on him. "Things like I don't bareback, I never fuck without condoms, I am a pushy bottom, and I don't have a gag reflex?"

"Damn, boy." Dolton had to grab his dick and squeeze. Dean was going to have him popping off before he touched him. "That is good to know, but I was talking about me." He stepped closer, inhaling the rich smells of sweat and man that poured from Dean, making his hunger worse. "I am a demanding top in bed but I will put out for the right man. I never fuck without condoms either, that's just stupid, and I have a huge dominant streak."

"God, fuck me," Dean moaned reaching out and caressing Dolton's chest. Fire travelled in the wake of his touch and Dolton growled.

"Soon, boy. But I need to know if this is what you want? I am not a sadist though if you need pain to get off, I can do that. What I want is to have you and your pleasure completely in my control. Do you want that, Dean? Because I have been fantasising about laying you out over my furs, holding your legs over your head and breeding your ass good."

"Damn, I want that, sir," Dean breathed. "I have a submissive streak, if you can tell." He chuckled.

"Like I didn't notice you jumping to when I told you to get in here."

"Then I want that, sir." Dean stepped in closer, whipping his shirt over his head, facing Dolton, dignity and submission in his stance. "You have my consent."

"And I am hung like a horse."

"Even better."

There was nothing left to say. Dolton practically ripped the remaining clothing off Dean and tossed his own somewhere behind him.

Damn, Dean was built. Broad shoulders, a firm muscled chest, slim hips and thick thighs—plus he had not been left behind when thick pretty cocks were handed out. His was pale at the base with a fat, purple, plum-shaped head. His body hair was nearly invisible save for the neatly trimmed patch surrounding the base of his dick.

Dolton paused in his efforts to catalogue every part of the man to let Dean run his appreciative eyes over his body. It had been a while since he had allowed anyone such close scrutiny of his body and he found that he enjoyed the attention.

"May I?" Dean questioned, moving in closer, his dick so swollen it was flat against his stomach and dripping like a faucet. Dolton looked down at his own body and knew that Dean was speaking of the tattoos that were etched into his body. "They are so beautiful…"

Dolton nodded and spread his arms wide, his own dick hanging low against his thigh. Dean ran his fingers over the tribal band of triangles and intricate spirals that encircled his left bicep.

"Huaorani tribe in the Amazon," Dolton explained, his voice going darker as Dean brushed gentle fingers over his skin. Dean's hand travelled across his shoulder to his chest and down to one dark nipple pierced with a golden hoop. "Africa, a Maasai tribesman gave it to me after I helped round up his cows after a lion attack."

Dean's eyes jerked to his and he bit his lower lip. "I can almost imagine you in beads and a kilt, chasing cows away from stalking lions."

"I was young and stupid," Dolton explained. "Invincible."

"And the scar?" Dean asked, touching a bit of raised skin on his left shoulder.

"Misunderstanding with a man holding a knife." Dean looked startled, but Dolton shook his head. "You should see what the other guy looked like."

After that, Dean made a game of guessing where the tat or body ornamentation came from. But when Dolton spun around, Dean appeared to be struck mute.

Across the skin of his back and down to the top of his ass, Dolton knew what his lover was seeing. There, in beautiful black and grey with red accents, rested a fierce scaled dragon blowing fire down his side while he shadowed a warrior figure dressed in black.

"Japan." Dolton laughed as Dean tried to stammer his questions. "I was young and stupid and picked a bar fight with a young Yakuza. Luckily for me his father was rather high-placed and wanted to teach his son a lesson in humility. When the gaijin darkie with the worst accent he had ever heard handed him his ass and apologised to the barkeep for destroying property, the man introduced himself. He was my sponsor for the short time on my first trip to Japan on my own. The man admired my intelligence and when I left he offered this tattoo as a remembrance."

"And you took it?"

"No one says no to the *kumicho*, the patriarch, when he offers an gift. It would be a grave insult." He turned back around and chuckled as Dean's eyes ran over his body once more. "You are beautiful, you know," he said in a matter-of-fact voice. "I am damn lucky to have you in my bed."

Dean didn't blush but his look turned so hungry that Dolton leaned in to press a soft kiss to his mouth, his tongue laving his full lip before pulling back with a soft nibble.

"You hit the genetic lottery, sir, and you know it." Dean snorted, shaking his head at him. "And you get the dick of death too."

"So how about we put it to good use?"

Nothing more needed to be said as they took to the shower.

As the hot water cascaded over Dean, darkening his hair to a deep brown, Dolton ran his hands over his new lover's body, grinning when Dean's nipples hardened into peaks as he pinched them.

"Harder," Dean demanded, leaning back against him. "I want to feel this next week."

"When I say so, boy." Dolton left his nipples alone to reach down and grip his dick. Dean gave a mewling hiss as he tightened his grip almost painfully. He backed off when Dean lolled against him in submission, at least for now.

He reached for his body wash and worked up a good lather before barking, "Face the wall," to Dean, his dick lurching as Dean readily complied. "So damn eager for what I got."

"Been wanting you for a long time, sir," Dean panted, his voice sounding harsh with arousal.

"We'll get there," Dolton offered as he began to thoroughly wash his lover down.

Dean's ass quivered, those two bubbles trembling when Dolton ran soapy thumbs down his trench to his hole. He then played with the soft globes of his ass, giving his flesh a firm squeeze just to hear Dean moan.

"You like having your ass played with?"

"I fucking love it," Dean panted, looking over his shoulder at him, his mouth slack, and his eyes at half-mast. "Can't wait to get you in there."

"Fuck," Dolton growled and began to swiftly clean his boy.

He dropped to his knees, spinning Dean around and taking the plump head of his cock into his mouth for a few quick slurps, getting his flavour before letting him go with a wet plop. Dean nearly screamed as his bright pink balls drew up, ready to unload. But Dolton gripped them, pulling them down as he rose to his feet.

From a shower rack, he pulled a small bottle of shampoo and lathered Dean's hair, running his finger thought the thick silk.

"I am going to have so much fun playing with this," he intoned, as he pushed Dean under the warm cascading water before he swiftly washed his own body. "Almost as much fun as I'm going to have playing with your pretty pink dick."

Dean was pulled out onto the shower mat and carefully dried with a thick towel. Then Dolton was leading him towards that round bed and the warm furs that waited for them. Dolton pushed his lover down and couldn't help but give his dick a few strokes as Dean settled back in the furs.

"Fuck, you're beautiful," he groaned when Dean pressed his feet flat to the bed and spread his legs wide, exposing his hungry hole and his seeping cock to his gaze. "Turn over."

Dean scrambled to go face down on the furs, gasping a soft, "Fuck," as he began working his dick through the softness there. Dolton watched his bubble butt flex and quiver as he ground his cock into the fur before leaning over and delivering a sharp slap, feeling a rush of possession flow thought him as his hand print blossomed bright red before fading into a sweet pink. "Stop that. That dick is for my pleasure."

"Sorry, sir." Dean looked up at him from beneath his long damp hair, looking as seductive as hell while waggling his ass at him. "Is this better?"

"Submissive my ass," Dolton snorted before crawling across the bed to loom over him.

"I told you I was demanding."

"And I told you I would make you beg—" He broke off as he parted those perfect buns and exposed his pink winking hole. "So fucking pretty," Dolton praised before he dived in.

Dean let out a squeal as Dolton hungrily began to tongue his hole."Damn, baby." Dolton pulled back and ran his tongue over the soft smooth skin. "Easy there."

But Dean was pushing back, whimpering as he tried to fuck himself on his tongue. Dolton gave his ass another slap, making Dean cry out sharply before he stilled.

"Better," Dolton praised, rubbing at the red handprint. He knew he would place more of them on his ass before this session was done. He loomed over Dean, pressing his chest to his back, letting him feel the heat and length of his muscles before pushing him face first into the furs. "Now stay there," he breathed into Dean's ear, feeling his body straining to remain still. "Let me enjoy this fine ass."

This time he shoved Dean's long hair off to the side and began to bite and lick at his neck.

"Please," Dean begged, as he buried his face in the furs. "Fuck, Sir!"

Dolton pressed a quick kiss to his neck before making his way down his boy's tender flesh.

Dean felt hot and firm beneath his hands, a perfect body to carry around the ass he so admired. When he reached it, he took his time, kneading it, playing with it before he spread those tempting cheeks wide. Dean's pink hole beckoned.

"Oh fuck!" Dean gasped as Dolton carefully lapped at the outer ring of muscle before taking a gentle bite. "Fuck, Dolton!"

"Hush," Dolton admonished, "I'm trying to enjoy my meal."

Dean tasted of soap and the heavier musk of man. It was a flavour he knew he was going to crave. He wanted to reach down and stroke his own dick, but he still wanted easy access to Dean's ass. So he would do the logical thing. "Reach back and spread them, boy."

Dan looked back at him, his face flushed with pleasure, his full lips redder than usual.

"That's right. Spread it open for me."

Eagerly Dean reached back and opened his own ass for Dolton.

"So pretty, baby," he complimented as he gripped his own dark dick in his hands and began leisurely to stroke himself. He lowered his head again and nipped at Dean's fingers before he began to lick him out in earnest.

"Sir—oh, sir," Dean moaned, writhing all over the bed but holding his own ass open for his sir's pleasure. "Fuck—I'm going to come."

"Not unless you can get it up again real fast," Dolton growled and shoved his tongue inside the tight muscle to caress the soft pink walls inside.

Dean wailed, his hips arching up sharply, and Dolton fought the urge to just shove his way inside.

Instead he pulled away—"Sir!"

"Just hold it open for me," Dolton ordered. "I want to see that hungry little hole winking at me." He kept his eyes on his lover, watching as his spit-wet asshole pulsed as Dolton moved to a shelf to remove condoms and some lube. "When was the last time you got good and fucked?"

His words made Dean visibly jump in anticipation as he rose up on his knees, still holding his cheeks apart for his sir's enjoyment.

"Years," he gritted out. "And I'm so hungry for it. Please, sir—fill me."

Dolton stalked back to the bed, tossing the lube and strip of condoms beside Dean's hips.

"You never answered my question," he reminded him. "On your knees or on your back?"

"Knees, sir," Dean answered, "But please, sir, please, can I touch you?"

Dolton's cock almost exploded as he imagined those hard callused hands caressing his body.

This was a body that routinely ploughed into men twice his size, knocking them on their asses and flattening the hell out of them. And now it was spread out for his pleasure, obeying his every command and wanting to service him. Dolton was blessed.

"Touch me, boy," he ordered, lying back on the bed, crossing his arms behind his head.

In a flash, Dean was on him, his lips pulling at his nipple ring, tugging his left nipple until he hissed pleasure, his chest arching towards the pleasure/pain.

Dean clamoured on top of him, his strong hand testing his strength as they tried to push him back into the furs. But Dolton reached up and gripped a handful of his hair, pulling him down to devour his mouth, their tongues duelling in a powerful wet kiss. He let him go when they both were breathless, sweating and straining against one another. "It's not going to suck itself." Dolton pointed to his cock that rose from his groin hot and hard.

In an instant Dean was on him, his cool damp hair caressing over Dolton's heated skin as he gripped the base of his cock.

"Fucking monster," Dean panted, looking dazed as he began to lap at the tip.

Dolton groaned and lay back as his lover's rough tongue slid over the throbbing head of his dick, lapping up the clear pre-cum.

"Yeah," he breathed, closing his eyes. "Keep going, baby. You know you want to."

One of Dean's hands went to his own cock as he gently sucked the head of Dolton's cock into his mouth.

"Damn, baby." Dolton felt the hot cavern of his mouth as his tongue, now soft and gentle, began to tease at his perineum, before he began sucking on the head.

"Fucking hot—wet—" Dolton gasped, forcing himself to lift his head and look. There, behind the curtain of damp blond hair, his lover's eyes stared contentedly up at him. Damn if his boy didn't love sucking cock. Dean was moaning around the dick in his mouth, one hand working rapidly between his legs, and he stroked his dick. He looked so hot Dolton had to close his eyes as he felt his balls began to rise.

Then Dean swallowed him to the base. Dolton blinked and looked down to be sure his eyes were sending his brain the correct signals. Then his baby swallowed and he thought the top of his head was going to explode.

"Fuck!" Dolton gasped as Dean pulled back, inhaling a quick breath with his nose, before he swallowed him whole, fucking his throat with Dolton's offered dick.

It was slick and tight, and as Dean swallowed around him, he found himself burying his hands in his lover's hair and fucking him faster. "Fuck, baby, you gonna make me come!"

The whining sounds Dean made were music to his sex-starved ears and as he felt his thighs tense up, as his nerves began shooting lightning through his back and spine, he knew he had to stop.

He used his hold on Dean's hair to pull him back before he pushed him face down on the furs.

"On your knees," he ordered, "Ass in the air. Lucky for you, this is not going to take long."

Dean eagerly assumed the position and threw his ass up in the air, waiting.

He slicked his fingers up and immediately eased one deep into his lover.

"Fuck, so good!" Dean groaned, pushing his ass back on his finger.

"So hungry," Dolton praised as his free hand ran over Dean's back, caressing his sides and watching as shivers overtook Dean's body. His hole opened beautifully for him, easily accepting his fingers. "You gonna gobble me up, baby?"

"Please, sir." He waggled his ass. "More."

"Soon," Dolton promised as he pulled his finger back before slicking up and adding a second.

Dean spread his legs wider as Dolton sank two fingers into his slick heat, his hips arching as he began to make small thrusts, fucking himself.

"Shh," Dolton soothed. "I'm going to stretch you out, baby. Pull you apart so I can fit inside."

"Please—I gotta have it! I need it—"

Dean was so hungry for his cock that it didn't take long at all before he was riding three fingers easily and begging for more.

Dolton pulled out, ignoring Dean's whine as he slicked up his cock and pulled on a condom. "I'm going to fuck the cum right out of you," Dolton promised. "Right now."

He placed one steadying hand on Dean's back before he spread his ass open wide. He pressed the head of his dick against the small pink opening that guarded his way into the paradise of Dean's body. He began to push in and felt the resistance as the guardian muscles struggled to open wide and accept his offering. Dean was growing tense, his shoulders tightening as he struggled to force his body to relax.

"Shh, baby," Dolton soothed. "Take it easy, boy. We got all night. I am not going to rush this."

He slid in steadily, feeling like his nuts were going to burst at the thought of being deep inside his lover's tight slick ass. He wanted in and he was going to get what he wanted.

He applied more pressure and suddenly Dean's hole opened up and pulled the head of his dick in.

"Shit!" Dean cried out and Dolton ran his hands over his ass, his thumbs spreading him wider as he praised his lover.

"So good, baby. You doing so very good—"

"Big," Dean panted. "Jesus!"

"You'll love it, baby. I promise."

"I've never had one this big—" He groaned as his ass spasmed, and Dolton had to force himself not to shove inside the strangling slick heat until he couldn't go any farther.

But this wasn't just some fuck. This was the object of his fantasies and Dean was going to be his baby for a long time, and if he wanted access to that sweet ass, he had better make sure he treated it right.

He began to rock slowly, feeling the tight pull of Dean's ass on his dick. After a few moments, Dean gave a shudder and his body opened up, sucking him in deep. But still he proceeded slowly, caressing his lover, hoping to ease his pain until the pleasure could commence.

Then Dean's pained whimpers turned into gasps as Dolton adjusted his angle and felt his shaft run along a bump that made his baby squeal.

"Right there!" Dean shouted, arching his back deeper and bouncing on his lover's dick slowly. "Hit it again, right there!"

"Is that hole hungry?" Dolton gripped his lover's cheeks and spread him wide, watching as the pink ring of muscle lapped out and around the base of his shaft. Dean pulled away and very carefully reversed his wiggle, his ass swallowing his dick again. "Come on, eat it up! Let that greedy little hole eat it all up—"

He pulled out and pushed forward, easing his dick in the hottest, sweetest place it had ever been.

"Fuck, sir!" Dean stammered, his movements smoothing out as he began to work his ass.

"Yeah, baby," Dolton gasped through gritted teeth, sweat rolling off his body. "So sexy—take it. Take it all—"

He leaned over and reached around Dean, his hands gripping his wet dick and getting a good hold. Dean shouted his approval and beginning to move faster. "Not going to last, sir!" Dean writhed. "Stroke my dick, Dol—Fuck! Stroke me hard!"

Using his pre-cum to ease the way, Dolton's fist began to fly over Dean's cock, flicking his thumb over the head and making the man rear back as his whole body quaked.

Dolton wrapped his free arm around his lover, pulling him back to his chest as he plucked at his nipples. Dean, his hair tangled and his red lips parted as his whole body flushed, rested his head on Dolton's shoulder.

"Mmm, sir," he moaned, held helplessly as Dolton began to thrust upwards, striking his prostrate on almost every thrust from the way he shook and his dick jumped in his hands. "Sir..." Dolton felt the nice slick sheath he was buried in began to tighten, milking his cock even as Dean stiffened in his arm. "Sir—I'm going to... Dolto—oh fuck! Gonna come! Gonna come!"

Dolton swooped down and took his lips, shoving his tongue in his mouth as he moved his fist faster, swallowing down Dean's screams as his body stiffened and his inner muscles began to milk his dick. Dean was coming and coming hard.

Dean tore his mouth away from Dolton's and threw his head back, bellowing his pleasure for the world to hear. His cock swelled to its fullest before it began to shoot slick streams of cum across Dolton's hand.

Dolton felt his lover tighten as his ass tried to strangle his cock.

He slowed his fist and his thrusts, easing Dean though his climax and pushing his body face first on the furs.

"I wanna feel it," Dean growled, turning his head to the side, one blue eye peering up at him through his hair.

It was enough to send him over the edge.

"Fuck!" he shouted as he slammed forward, burying all of his ten inches deep in his lover, his own hips pumping and grinding as he struggled to breed his baby. "Damn, Dean," he gasped as his balls slammed against the base of his cock and he could feel his seed shoot from his body to be caught in the condom.

Dean moaned and Dolton knew it was because he could feel the extra heat of his release filling the condom. His body stiffened and eased as the last of his seed pulsed from his cock.

"Damn, baby," he groaned, collapsing on his lover's back, neither minding that Dean was in the wet spot or that they were sweating all over each other. "Next time, the load is going over your back."

As he'd thought, there were no objections.

Later he would get them up and cleaned before he fed his new lover and laid him out on his bed to ready him to fuck again if his ass could take it.

Dean fit him like a glove and now that he had reached his goal of getting the man into his bed, his new objective was to keep him there.

Chapter Five

His phone ringing pulled Dean from a sexed-out doze. He glared at his cell for a moment before a heavy arm dropped over his stomach, urging him back into the heat of a hot muscular chest. Dolton Pride threw off heat like a furnace and was an unabashed snuggler. He glared at his lover, as he was the one who'd snagged their cell phones and placed his on the bedside table nearby, before relaxing into Dolton's sleepy embrace.

Dean looked up and noted two things, he was starving and the sun was shining again. He looked at his happily buzzing phone and wanted to smash it. Instead he reached for it, winching at the soreness in his ass.

Dolton had a monster cock and the skill to use it to draw happy screams from his throat. Problem was after the screaming was done, the soreness set in. His ass burned, not that it hurt hard enough to prevent him from doing it again. He just needed a few hours, a good breakfast, and he would be ready to go again. But the damn phone was still ringing.

Groaning, he reached out and snatched it up, waking Dolton in the process. He sighed when he saw who was calling and answered because he knew his friend would keep calling.

"Robbie," he snapped. "What the fuck do you want?" Dean was never in a good mood after being woken up and even worse if there was no coffee in his system.

"Good morning to you, sunshine." Robbie's voice annoyed the crap out of him.

"What," he enunciated very carefully, "do you want?"

"It's early so I thought I could come over and—"

"No."

"You didn't even know what I was going to ask."

"Doesn't matter. I'm not home."

"Well, shit," Robbie chucked. "You get laid last night or something?"

"Yes," Dean snapped. "And I need to sleep."

"Who you fucking?" Robbie sounded like he really wanted to know. "Anyone I know? The only woman I see you around is our coach, and I would have bet doughnuts to dollars that she was a ball-busting rug-muncher."

"Really?" Dean gritted out, relaxing a little when he felt Dolton move up behind him and start to nuzzle his neck. "Coach?" Dean pulled his cell away from his ear and stared down at the grinning picture of his former friend before he put it back to his ear. "Are you insane? I am not fucking Coach, Robbie. I respect the woman too much to hit on her."

This conversation was making Dean very angry and uncomfortable and all he wanted was food and sleep…and maybe more sex—he didn't care about the order. He needed Robbie off the phone.

"Well, she turned me down flat so she has to be a dyke. Besides, what woman would want to coach a football team?"

"We done?" Dean sighed, closing his eyes at his friend's stupidity. He just couldn't deal without caffeine in his system.

"Yeah, man. Call me this weekend when you pull yourself out of your pussy."

"Whatever," Dean grumbled, disconnecting the call before slamming his phone back onto the table.

"Your friend is an ass."

"You heard that?"

"Yup, and if Coach heard that she would have his balls for earrings. I do not mess with the Dragon Lady. She has powerful friends."

"Hmm." Dean slumped back to the bed and looked up as his lover hovered over him.

"Hungry?" Dolton asked, bending down to steal a kiss, unmindful of morning breath.

"A little," Dean admitted. "My ass hurts."

"It was hungry last night. I fed it."

"Too fucking much," Dean laughed, reaching up to pull Dolton back down into another kiss. Fuck morning breath. The man felt too good to let out of his arms.

"If your ass is hurting, I can run you a bath—"

Dean looked around the room and blushed as the memories of last night's debauchery began to flood into his mind.

Dolton, good as his word, cleaned him up and brought him down to his bed. Once here, he braided Dean's hair into a long tail that he wrapped in leather then used to tie him to the headboard.

With Dean's head unable to move, Dolton pulled out some silk straps and introduced him to the beautiful yet effective world of Shibari, Japanese rope bondage.

Dolton started light, knotting a cord around Dean's neck before training it between his legs, another knot behind his balls stimulating his prostate from the outside when the ropes were tightened or he shifted. His arms were lashed to his side in a corset-like tying that left his ass framed and pushed his dick out for presentation. Dean then was driven nearly out of his mind as his lover licked and bit at any exposed flesh.

His balls were swollen and purple, filled to overflowing by the time Dolton had taken him into his hot mouth. The man might have a gag reflex, but he knew how to give head like a pro. Dean was licked, sucked and nibbled until he literally was screaming for his lover to stop. Then he was flipped over as Dolton rediscovered the love of his ass.

"Such a pretty ass, baby," Dolton praised, running his hands over the quivering surface. He parted Dean's cheeks and spent many minutes playing with his hole, running his fingers over it, licking it, and finally reaching into his bedside table to open a new vibrator. It was swiftly covered in a condom, slicked up, and pressed into his hungry ass.

"Gotta keep you open and ready for me, baby," Dolton teased as he began to fuck him with the hard plastic.

It felt wicked and delicious, being spread open, the burning pain of entry, the thought of Dolton's golden eyes watching the silver fake dick slide in and out of his ass.

When Dolton turned the damn thing on, Dean was sure the neighbours were going to call the cops, thinking someone was being murdered. Dolton managed to find his prostate, his very sensitive and abused prostrate, and proceeded to dance the vibrator over it. Dolton pressed bites all over his ass, never enough to bruise or to mark, but enough to be an added sensation to the fire that was zinging through his body.

He was nearly in tears and begging to be filled as Dolton withdrew the vibrator and started with fingers again. Dolton was wiggling three in his ass before he gave up his play and wrapped his massive dick in a condom.

Dolton was roughly ten inches of thick cock and Dean's ass, especially after the extended foreplay, had gobbled up every fucking inch.

The second time was more intense as he could not move to take what he wanted. He had not been lying when he'd told Dolton that he was a demanding bottom. He had been known to flip over a top who was not giving the dick up properly and take what he needed. But Dolton was not like those guys. It was like something in him was innately alpha. Maybe it was his time spent proving his worthiness to be included in the different tribes he lived with during his studies or maybe it was just a part of him, but Dolton Pride was a sensual Dom down to his bones.

So while Dean struggled and finally gave in to the tight comfort of the ropes, Dolton had taken his time fucking his ass, drawing it out until he was so sensitive he could barely stand to feel the air on his flesh. That neat corset tie that held his dick front and centre also acted as a very effective cock ring. He was not getting off until Dolton allowed it.

He had begged, he had screamed and pleaded, but only when he went lax, giving his body over to Dolton's care, did Dolton allow him to come. And come he did. He blasted so hard, he nearly passed out.

He pulled himself together as Dolton unwound the ropes and surprise surprise, after a few moments, there wasn't even a mark to show what had been done to help turn his body out. But it left his asshole swollen, red and gaping.

Dolton ran him a bath in his huge Jacuzzi tub and soaked with him in Epsom Salt-treated water while feeding him slices of fruits and vegetables.

Dolton had thought of everything and Dean had never felt more cherished.

But now in the light of day, Robbie's unwelcome presence had come calling and now he was irritated, hungry and irritated.

"I know he's an ass," Dean grumbled. "But he didn't use to be that way. Something happened to change him."

"All I know is that the other guys are about tired of him and Coach is ready to hang a heel up his ass. The only reason he is still on the team is because they like to keep my right tackle happy," Dolton teased. "And my right tackle isn't happy unless he is knocking some lineman flat on his ass — or getting fucked."

"Try fed," Dean snorted. "I am all fucked out. This hole is closed for business."

"Pity," Dolton smirked before he dived beneath the covers. "But the dick is still open for business."

And who was he to complain about getting a world-class blow job? Dean just resigned himself and took one for the team. After all, it was what a good teammate did.

By the end of the weekend, Dean and Dolton had gone through two boxes of extra-large condoms and five tubes of flavoured lube, established that Dolton lived to rim, and learnt more about each other than anyone — except for their therapists who probably would not approve of the method used to get them talking.

Chapter Six

"I'm going to tell them."

"Don't do anything on my account," Dolton leered as he watched Dean squeeze into his tight athletic pants, his jock outlining that perfect ass he had plundered so much that he was amazed Dean still had the energy, let alone the strength, to walk. "I don't think the guys will care so much but you have your friend to think about."

Dolton looked around the empty locker room, glad for once that they'd arrived early. He could take the ribbing from his friends on the team if they commented on them arriving together. But he was liable to just punch Dean's friend in the jaw if one derogatory word passed his lips.

"Robbie's changed. He is not the same man I went to school with. I don't know, Dolton. It's so fucked up and wrong what he has become." Dean slammed his locker door closed, the sound echoing around the empty room, before staring at Dolton in confusion. "Something major had to have happened."

"Mmm." Dolton nodded. There was no doubting his point. Robbie Keton was all kinds of fucked up and wrong and rarely did a man become that way on his own.

"So no matter what I do, he'd find something to bitch about." Dean hefted his pads over his shoulders and began to lace them up firmly. "And I want to tell them. I want them to know what I managed to pick up in my spare time."

"Spare time, huh?" Dolton purred, stepping closer to his man as the other players began to file in. "I got something you can do with your spare time."

Instead of pulling away, Dean lunged forward, gripping Dolton by the shoulders, and attacked his mouth.

Dolton didn't pull away. Instead he dropped his hands to the ass he loved so well and pulled Dean in closer.

Dean broke off the kiss to hiss in startled pain and arousal and he stared up into Dolton's eyes.

"When we are done" — Dolton's words were low and precise — "I am going to take you back to my place, tie you to my bed, and fucking eat your ass until you come." He fisted one hand in Dean's abundant hair and jerked his head back. "And then I'm going to fuck you until you scream."

Dean made some kind of strangled noise but thrust his hips forward, his arousal pushing out the pocket of his bright blue jock.

"Yes, baby," Dolton purred, grinding back, hissing as his own erection pressed into Deans, grinding his cup into him and biting back a hiss because stimulation was stimulation and it had to hurt Dean the right way from the way the man closed his eyes and leaned into the pain. "You gonna give it all up to me?"

"What the fuck?"

The question was shouted with some outrage as Dolton tightened his grip on his trembling lover.

Slowly he turned from the lust-dazed face to stare at one Robbie Keton, his mouth hanging open, his bag over his shoulder, his pads gripped in one hand. The man had frozen where he stood, his eyes wide as he stared from one man to the other.

Dolton couldn't help it. He smirked at the man before lowering his head to take Dean's lips in a hard kiss.

Dean trembled and returned the kiss with just as much fervour, as if Robbie were not even there. Moaning his approval, Dolton thrust his tongue between his lover's lips and stole a quick taste before pulling back. Dean tasted of coffee, chocolate and his own spicy self.

"Move, man."

The shouted words turned Dolton's attention away from Dean and to the rapidly filling locker room. Apparently someone had objected to Robbie taking up space in the middle of the floor and holding up progress. They shoved him aside and still the man stared.

"The fuck? Dean? What the fuck, man? You fucking queer for Baldie?"

"The term is gay, Robbie." Dean shook himself as he gained control and turned to face his friend. "Homosexual if you want to get politically correct."

"You fucking him? Jesus!" Robbie threw his pads down and began to pace, the other players filing in, some ignoring the whole affair and going about their business of suiting up while a few others stood around watching this new bullshit unfold.

"No." Dolton recognised the anger in Dean and took a step back, letting the man handle his own battles.

"Not at all." Dean turned towards Robbie and shot the whole room a baleful glare. "He's fucking me."

"Bastard!" Robbie shouted, slamming his shit to the ground and charging Dean.

But he didn't get very far. As Dolton pushed his lover aside, ready to defend him, several of the players grabbed Robbie, holding the struggling man back.

"Oh, fuck you, Robbie." Dean stepped around Dolton and Dolton held his hands up, letting the man do as he wished. If Dean wanted to kick the bastard's ass, it was on him. But Dolton would be sure to have his back. So he crossed his arms and waited as the shouting grew louder.

"None of your fucking business," someone— sounded like Aiden Brewer—roared, narrowing his eyes as he glared at Robbie.

"But he's a fucking fag!" Robbie shouted. "That shit ain't right!"

"Obviously you've never been in the locker room after a good game."

The new feminine voice had them all turning to stare at the petite figure of Coach as she stormed into the locker room, uncaring about the partial nudity around her. Her narrowed eyes took in the aggressive stance of the men before she started to speak.

"Gentlemen." Her piercing gaze moved over her players. "Save it for the fucking field. Am I clear?"

As Coach was the one person to organise the team, fund the team, and come up with some damn good plays that kept them in top form, the men respected her. They loved her for her no-nonsense approach to keeping the Griffins on top.

"You can't allow this to happen!" Robbie turned towards her, his anger still apparent as his face turned a brilliant shade of red and his fists clenched at his side. "This shit ain't right."

"Who's to say what's right and what's wrong, Mr Keton? I didn't bring you on to be the moral police. I brought you on to keep the other fucking guys off my quarterback. Do your fucking job and save the sermon for Sunday's meeting. You are here to play a game. Protect my fucking quarterback, Mr Keton. That's all I give a fuck about."

"Fucking dyke," Robbie growled and the whole room went silent.

Coach turned smartly on her bright red heels and smirked at Robbie. "Wouldn't you like to know?" she purred. "Or am I a dyke because you will never fucking ever find out?"

The laughter at her statement made Robbie flush even further, though he was no longer huffing like a bull.

"Now do your job. Protect my quarterback and then we can talk about your future with the Griffins."

With Coach's departure, chatter once again filled the locker room. Dolton looked over at Dean and instead of looking upset, the man looked relieved and agitated as hell.

"This isn't over," Robbie snapped, bending to heft his equipment.

"As far as I am concerned, yes, it is," Dean replied, rolling his eyes, and he ran his hands through his long hair.

"So much fucking goes on around here, you have to be blind to miss it," Aiden added, smirking at someone across the room.

"We could sell tickets and get our funding for the next two years," someone else interjected to the laughter of many.

The players went about their business, suiting up for the game joking about the newest explosion.

"You okay?" Dolton asked as Robbie stalked to his locker.

"I can take care of myself." Dean glared at him.

"I know that." Dolton raised both hands in a placating manner. "I was just, you know, having your back."

Dean blew hard, staring at him for a moment, before turning away.

"Hey." Dolton reached for him, gripping him by the arm and turning Dean to face him again. "Hey —"

"I said I could fight my own battles."

"And I told you that I know that," Dolton countered. "I just want you to know that you are not alone."

"This is not the wilds of Outer Mongolia," Dean snapped. "Nor am I some innocent tribesman who needs to be protected from the great white plague —"

"I never said that."

"But you sure are acting it."

"I am a man of action." Dolton was frowning now, staring down at Dean like he had grown another head. What the fuck was wrong with his lover? "I couldn't stand by and do nothing while you were being attacked."

"Yeah, well, maybe I don't need you to be my fucking shield, Dolton. I mean — fuck! I can handle myself."

"I know that," Dolton growled and Dean shivered, his eyes growing wide at the familiar bass in his voice. "You could probably kick my ass."

"Why would I kick it when I want to fuck it?"

Oh, Dolton thought to himself. *That is what this new outburst is about.*

"You want to fuck my ass, Blondie?"

"Yeah, I do." Dean took a step forward, getting in his face. "I think it's time you bent over for me."

Dolton jumped as he felt Dean's hand connect with his ass sharply, sending a flood of adrenaline through his body.

"Oh yeah?" Dolton breathed, bending down, wanting nothing more than to kiss that smug look off his face.

"After the game." Dean turned and walked away, leaving a stunned Dolton staring hungrily at his ass while some of his teammates laughed their asses off at his predicament. He looked down and winced as his swelling dick nearly shoved outside of his cup.

"Gonna scare some Dragons with that package?" some wiseass shouted out, making the room erupt in more laughter.

"Fuck you all!" Dolton called out, laughter in his own voice as his own sense of humour saw the delicious irony in his situation. There he was, the master, being taken down a peg by quiet unassuming Dean — and he loved it.

"Don't think you have the strength for that," someone answered, leaving him to flip off the room as he turned to his locker to finish getting ready.

Damn, he was going to make his baby boy pay...right before he let him fuck his ass into next week. His hole twitched hungrily thinking about it. It had been some time since he'd bottomed and he could hardly wait for the game to be over to feel the burn of Dean's pretty cock stretching him out and taking him hard.

It was going to be a long four quarters.

Chapter Seven

"Huddle up!" The Griffins' quarterback called his defenders to crowd around and began to swiftly go over the play.

"It's second and seven. I want to run a long play here. We got the time. I am going to fake a pass to Rodriguez to buy us some time. Rogers and Bentley, break free and go long. One of you will be my target. Pride, Majors, and Keton, keep your eyes open. The Dragons are out for my blood and I can't have my pocket break down before I can get the ball out. And if I fumble, for the love of God, recover the ball."

"Some of us are better at grabbing balls than others," Robbie drawled and blinked at the sudden silence that fell.

"Aggression is good," the quarterback snapped, glaring at him from between the face shield of his helmet. "But save it for the Dragons. On three—break!"

The defensive line went all hands in for the shake and raced to take their spots before a delay of game penalty could be called.

"So…this why you can't keep in touch with your old friend?" Robbie snarled as Dean bent over and took his position, sizing up the player opposite to him. "You too busy getting fucked by the nerd?"

"Not the place," Dean snapped and tried to put his full concentration on his own target. The huge linebacker facing him grinned.

"Gonna knock you on your ass, baby! Whoo!" the man shouted and Dean smirked. He could take this bastard. It was going to be so effin' easy.

There was the snap and Dean sprang into action, slamming into his target, shoving the larger man flat on his back while his momentum carried him further, taking out another tackle, and giving his quarterback time to set up the throw.

He was scrambling back to his feet, looking to take someone else out when a jarring pain hit his left side, nearly knocking the breath out of him.

He rolled with the fall, landing on his back to see Robbie lying against him.

"Sorry, bro," he sneered. "You got in my way."

Before he could say anything else, the whistle was blowing and he turned his head enough to see that Bentley had got the ball and ran it in for a touchdown.

Then the others were converging, gripping his hands and pulling him to his feet. The many congratulatory ass smacks he got were making his cock ache. His hard-on from teasing Dolton earlier had never really gone away. And now with the adrenaline rush—he looked away and tried to picture Coach naked and fucking the green and black Griffins' mascot. It was enough to scare the blood back to his brain.

As special teams took the field, he whipped off his helmet and struggled to walk normally to the sidelines. He jerked and turned as he got one final slap that felt more like a caress. He looked over to see

Dolton walking beside him, helmet dangling from his fingers.

"Nice stop," the man drawled and Dean grunted as his cock filled once more. He looked down at his dick then up at his lover, a smirk pulling at his lips.

"You are so going to suck my dick after this—"

"Gonna swallow you whole, baby." Dolton's eyes grew dark and hungry as he stared at him. "Then if you are real good, you get a shot at my ass."

Then he abruptly spun around and watched as Paul Toth smoothly kicked for three. The crowd went wild and thus paid no attention to the linebacker quietly adjusting his cock.

"You think you so cute," Dolton casually remarked and Dean didn't even bother to hold in his groan of irritation.

"You're right." He nodded, running his hands though his loose hair. It would be a tangled mess by the time the game was done, but he loved the feel of it hanging down over the back of his jersey. "Though my boyfriend calls me beautiful." He chuckled as Dolton flipped him off as he walked over towards the water table.

"When did you turn queer?" Robbie asked, ignoring the hustle as the offensive team took to the field. "What made you that way?"

"I was always this way, Robbie," Dean turned to stare at him, shaking his head sadly. What the hell had become of his friend? The proud and arrogant young man who tolerated everyone around him even if he didn't exactly accept them had been replaced by a balding, overweight asshole of an ageing jock with a god-complex. It was sad. "You don't turn gay. You are or you aren't."

"Did you ever—" He looked self-conscious and kind of green and Dean fought the urge to vomit when he realised where this conversation was going.

"Oh hell no, Robbie. We are not having this conversation."

"You spent nights—"

"You are so not my type." Dean grimaced. "That thought of seeing you naked... Ugh, no, man. Just no."

"What's wrong with me?" Suddenly the snarling bear was back and Dean rolled his eyes, used to Robbie's swift shifts in mood.

"Really? You want to have this conversation now?" He stepped closer, noting with some satisfaction that Robbie took a step back. "Because I have a whole fucking list of shit that's wrong with you—starting with your attitude."

Wisely, Robbie backed off and Dean huffed as he spun away and stormed over to the benches.

"Your friend is a real piece of work."

Dean looked up to see Dolton handing him his water bottle. He grunted and snatched it away, tossing his head back and taking a long pull.

He peered over at his lover and noted that heavier breathing and the way his eyes were glued to his throat and trailed his eyes down to his crotch.

"Looks like little Dolton wants to come out and play." He grinned at Dolton's frown.

"Who said anything about little?"

Dean just smirked and scooted over as Dolton collapsed next to him. "Really, Robbie Keton is a dick."

"He didn't used to be this way." Dean shrugged, leaning forward so his elbows rested on his knees before eyeing his lover carefully. "Something must have happened to change him."

"Or he was a dick all along and something brought it out in him."

"True." He turned his head to watch Robbie storm over to the water cooler before speaking softly. "But he's not who I want to talk about now."

"Is that so?"

"That is very much so, sir." Dean cut his eyes back to his lover and watched as a dark red flush ran up his face. "I want to talk about how I want to spread your cheeks and eat you out real slow."

He had to hold in a chuckle as Dolton swallowed hard and quickly looked away.

"I want to make you beg, sir. I want to make you beg and plead, and scream for me. Then I'm going to push in slowly, stretching you out before I pound you. That is what I want to talk about."

"You are so going to pay for this," Dolton murmured, spreading his thighs and showing his bulging crotch. His pants and jock were barely containing his straining dick.

"I certainly hope so —"

"Let's move!" Dean blinked as their cosy little bubble of lust popped as Coach's abrasive voice called for her defensive line.

"Later," Dolton promised, his voice dark as sin as he slammed his helmet on his head and strutted out to the field.

After shaking his head, Deal donned his own helmet and followed, praying that all this teasing would net him the opportunity to sink his dick into his lover's fine ass.

* * * *

"Dragons' defence is killing us," the quarterback muttered as he called his team together. They were down by three and at this point his only goal was to get the ball down field close enough for a shot at the uprights. "I am going to Bentley this time," he called the audible. "Pride, Majors, Brewer, I am counting on you guys to get me some time for this long drive. Keton, remember," he added sarcastically, "save it for the other team. The green and black are our guys."

Robbie snorted and Dolton eyed the man carefully. He was up to something. He had been taking pot shots and small dives at Dean all game long. If he were going to do something, now would be the time when they were deep in the last minutes of the fourth quarter. He wouldn't be able to do anything in the locker rooms and he appeared to be too much of a coward to try something after the game.

Despite his lover's objections, he was keeping an eye on Dean. Robbie had done nothing overt, but Dolton had seen this behaviour before. Once while he was in the Amazon within a remote settlement of the Huaorani of Ecuador, he had observed one of their young men, a young warrior, eyeing him suspiciously. He had tried not to take offence, knowing that 'civilised' society had done much to destroy the culture and way of life of this tribe. So he had mostly ignored it.

When at spear practice, for the Huaorani were still mainly a hunter-gatherer society, if a spear had come too close it was just bad luck. When he had climbed to the treetop bower that the jaguar worshipers allowed for his use and the ties that held the floor in place gave way, he had chalked it up to age. And if he had not been able to find his way back to the settlement after a hunt when something obliterated his markings, he had called it the work of a territorial animal. But when he was on his last days, when they were having a war dance in his honour, the young warrior had struck, leaping at him from beneath a cover of leaves and trees and trying to drive a knife into his back.

He had walked away from that situation with a new scar on his shoulder from the blade's first slash, the title of warrior for showing restraint in just kicking the young punk's ass instead of outright killing him, and the new ability to observe suspect behaviour. Robbie was acting about as suspect as they came.

As they took their positions on the field, Dolton's attention was torn between the offensive lineman before him and the traitorous linebacker on his line.

"Seventeen! Fifteen! Twenty-three! Hike!"

The ball was snapped and Dolton charged at his target, keeping one eye on Dean and stealing glances at Robbie.

It was when his full attention was lax, after he was standing over the lineman he flattened, that Robbie struck. But instead of going after Dean like he expected, Robbie went straight for him.

He felt the impact on his side as the air was driven from his mouth. A hand came up and he felt his head snap back as an elbow slammed his chin up, sending his helmet flying.

A red haze darkened his eyesight as pain washed over him, tipping his already adrenaline-drenched nerves into overdrive.

With a roar, he reached for the thing causing him pain, got a good grip, wrapped his legs around it and flipped so that he was on top of the enemy. Then he was tucking his head low to protect his neck and raining down blows on the writhing thing that dared attack him.

Then there was screaming and whistles shrilling and many hands trying to pull him away. Yellow things, flags he realised as he calmed, were fluttering around him and he looked down to where he was seriously trying to fuck up one shocked Robbie Keton.

The man's helmet was gone and his watery blue eyes looked up at him in shock as blood ran down his nose and smeared across his face.

"—the fuck is wrong with you?" That was Coach screaming at them both and as he allowed his teammates to pull him back, he realised that he was not getting yelled at. Robbie was flat on his back, their team surrounding them, as the officials began making announcements.

"Foul unnecessary roughness, fifteen-yard penalty — Griffins."

"You got a fucking penalty fighting with your own team? Jeeeesus! What the fuck is wrong with you? Out! You are out of the game!"

Even Dolton winced as Coach unleashed her fury upon the downed man. She turned to Dolton and he flinched. He had not lost control that badly since he had got into a bar-room brawl with a group of Yakuza when he was young and cocky the first time he was in Japan.

She looked him up and down and it was then he noticed the taste of blood in his mouth. He had bitten his tongue sometime during the fight, and the pain, along with his other aches, were only now making themselves known.

"Nice moves," she smirked before turning and making her way off the field, her scarlet red cross-trainers replacing the heels that she typically wore.

He looked up and recognised Dean's stiff face as he held a hand out for him. Shaking his head, he took it and was not surprised in the strength of the other man as he practically jerked him to his feet.

Dean reached up and tilted his head down to examine his face before he turned to face Robbie who was struggling to his feet.

He took one step before Dolton realised what he was doing and wrapped his arms around his chest, holding him in place.

"Now is not the time," he muttered, patting him on the chest as the team began to leave the field.

"Son of a bitch," someone bellowed as Dolton retrieved his helmet and looked around. The ball, which had been carried down to the thirty-fifth-yard line and a doable kick, was now moved back to the fiftieth and a difficult shot for Paul to make.

They were at the fourth and had no choice but to try to get the ball through the goal to tie the score.

Everyone took position to protect the kicker and a hush fell over the field. The eerie silence remained as Paul lined up and the ball was snapped. The holder got the ball in place as Dolton and the defensive line did their best to give Paul enough time to set up properly.

Dolton was on the ground when he heard Paul's foot connect with the ball. He flipped over to his back, ignoring the soreness in his side, as he watched the ball soar high in the air. The red pigskin spiralled as it flew clear and true towards the uprights—veering to the left—then tipping to the left bar, tagging it with a sharp metallic thwap and falling outside of the line.

"Fuck!" Dolton shouted as his team members groaned their defeat. The kick was no good. The Griffins had lost.

Chapter Eight

"What the fuck, man?" Dolton couldn't stop himself from slamming Robbie against his locker as soon as he saw the other man. He jammed his forearm under Robbie's throat, forcing his head up, his eyes to his as Dolton awaited his answer.

The other members of the team stood back and watched or stormed towards their lockers, but anger was the prevalent emotion in the room. No one even thought to help Robbie Keton.

"Let me go!" Robbie ordered, his breath heaving, his eyes wide, as spittle flew from his mouth. He had been cleaned up since he was ejected from the game and now a neat white bandage covered a hopefully broken nose. "I am so going to fucking sue you."

"Not if he sues you first." In the commotion, no one had noticed the click of red heels as Coach made her way into the room. "And I so fucking hope he does."

An arm on his shoulder made Dolton stand down as soon as he realised it was his lover pulling him back in control. He stepped back and glared at Robbie, remaining in a ready stance.

"He attacked me!"

"After you gave him an illegal hit that was so bad that the officials penalised us! You got penalised for a personal foul on one of your own teammates. What the hell were you thinking?"

"I was thinking that he turned my buddy queer!"

At his words anger turned into disgust as the team members began to file away in droves.

"Half this whole fucking team is queer!" Coach shouted, looking angrier by the second. "Are you blind or are you just stupid?"

Robbie looked around at the men he had been playing with, the men he had showered with, the men he had shared camaraderie and beer and bullshit with. "I think I'm going to vomit."

"Good," Coach snorted. "And when you're done, clean out your locker."

"Wh—"

"Do you really think that anyone here trusts you now?"

"But I was NFL—"

"And right about now that and a buck might get you a cup of coffee. We don't need players who turn on their own. Drop off your uniform, gather your shit and get the fuck out."

"And you are going to make me go?" Trying to save face, Robbie stepped forward, posturing heavily as he tried to stare down the petite Asian woman. Before he could take another step, Dean was stepping forward, violently shoving his friend back.

"What the fuck is wrong with you, Robbie? You didn't used to be this way. I mean, what the fuck, man?"

There was silence as Coach shook her head and turned to face her players.

"This game was lost through no fault of our own. In my eyes that makes us champions, though the footage speaks for itself. So this is what we are going to do. We are going to practise harder, fight harder, and we will never let anything like this affect our solidarity again." She looked around at the men and it felt as if her gaze were sizing them up, daring them to call her words a lie. "We are brothers, united in our efforts to win this thing. We won't let anything, not despair, not anger, not resentment...not even fucking providence keep us from what is rightfully ours!" There were shouts of agreement and some catcalls, but Coach's brightly painted red lips pulled up in a mean sneer. "We will face the Dragons again, and as Dragons are natural enemies of Griffins, the war will be bloody and the battle will be hard. But remember. Dragons went extinct way before Griffins."

She smirked as most of the team ignored Robbie and began to cheer. All around him, men in various states of undress were slapping each other's hands, pumping their fists in the air, rebuilding a bond that had been bruised, but not destroyed, by the one who was now an outsider. "Griffins do more than fly, gentleman. We soar! And we will soar again in three weeks' time when we put those Dragons back in their caves and seal the fucking doors!"

The cheers were deafening, echoing around the locker room that had seen so much action, witnessed so many tears, so much heartbreak and triumph.

Coach turned and strode out of the room, the sound of her heels lost in the resounding cheers as the team slowly began to lick their wounds and pull themselves back together as a cohesive group.

Soon after, the men began to leave, some in groups, some alone, but all with a sense of accomplishment.

The showers turned on and the air became humid with the smell of sweat and men.

Dolton looked around and realised that he was standing in the midst of a closed tribe, as it were. And he was thick in the middle of it.

He had witnessed an interloper making his way into the group, watched as he created tension with his posturing, trying to take the alpha spot. He had seen cultures clash as the interloper realised that though this group was matriarchal and like the Huaorani, hadn't really had any one leader, though the appropriate people stepped up to take the lead when their particular skillset was needed. He had watched and even participated as dissension had turned into derision as the interloper realised he could not sway people to his way of thinking and tempers exploded in a high-stress environment. And right now, he had watched the matriarch step up and claim leadership long enough to further unite the group before leaving them feeling stronger as a whole.

He turned to look at his lover and frowned when he saw him staring at the interloper, at Robbie, anger still painting his face.

They stood there glaring at each other for God knew how long as players gathered their things and after casting pitying looks at Robbie left for celebrations and reconnections of their own. Finally it was only the three still standing there, tension building in the air. It cracked a little as Dean spoke again to his once childhood friend.

"What happened to you?"

"You don't understand!" Robbie shouted back. "You don't. You sit here with your business and your geek friends" — he glared at Dolton but was wary enough not to approach the man — "being all perfect and shit with your long blond hair. You don't know how it is, man. You can't understand."

Realising that the posturing was all done but for the submissive whining that was sure to follow, Dolton turned to his lover, dismissively putting his back to Robbie as if the man had ceased to exist to him. And in a way, he had. The broken man was of no concern to him, and as Dean stated, he could handle himself. "Are you going to be okay?"

"Yeah." Dean ran his hands thought his hair, shaking his head while staring at his ex-friend because Dolton knew there was no way Dean would ever welcome his ass back into their fold. "I'll be fine."

"You wanna get out of here?"

"I want—to talk to Robbie," Dean breathed, turning his attention fully on Dolton. "Why don't you get cleaned up and wait for me. If we go back to your place, I want to use your hot tub...so long as we still have plans?"

Despite his anger and soreness, Dolton allowed a wicked grin to cross his face. He leaned in and whispered, "You can fuck my ass all you want, tough guy. You have more than earned the right."

He reached around, not caring about his audience at all, and cupped Dean's ass, feeling the tight muscle and the soft skin...feeling the perfect bubble butt quiver as he reaffirmed his possession. His dick jumped to attention and he knew even after he got fucked, he was going to sink his hard inches into his lover before the day ended.

Dean growled before gripping Dolton by the shoulders and jerking him up to his level. Then Dean's mouth was covering his, his tongue invading as Dolton pushed back, teasing, tasting and savouring the flavour of his lover.

"Thirty minutes." Dolton pulled back and growled at him. "You got thirty minutes then I am walking out of here. And if you are not with me, I am going home, greasing up my dildo and fucking myself raw. You can watch."

He turned as Dean's groan filled the still air while he moved to his locker and snatched up his bag. Pads and the rest could be removed in the shower. His side hurt, but nothing a few aspirin and some hot water wouldn't take care of. Then he would get his lover home and slowly take him apart with sex. It was decadent, hedonistic, and he could hardly wait.

* * * *

Turning back to Robbie, Dean shook his head as he stared at the shattered remains of his once friend. *How the mighty have fallen*, he thought uncharitably before shaking that nonsense from his head.

"How could you—" Robbie started but Dean cut him off.

"Easy. I spread my legs and demand to be filled."

Robbie blanched, the flush of anger on his face fading away until he looked sickly and pale, the bruises on his face already setting in.

"You—a fag—"

"I prefer the term gay. Queer is a cute word too, Robbie, but I really like gay. It explains why I am so fucking happy."

"Happy—"

"Don't I look fucking happy?" Dean roared, his anger getting the better of him for a moment. "Jesus, Robbie! I bring you here in good faith, I support you when none of your NFL buddies can stand to be around you, I get you in good with my team and you fucking attack one of our own? What the fuck is wrong with you?"

"You wouldn't understand—"

"Then how about you explain it quickly. I got a date in half an hour and I refuse to miss it."

Robbie foundered for a moment, as if he didn't expect Dean to allow him to speak so he didn't quite know what to say.

"Well?" Dean snapped impatiently.

"It's—God…"

"I'm out of here." At the first hint of religion, Dean turned and made for his locker. He had made peace with God a long time ago and his God didn't condemn love. His God *was* love.

"Dean—"

"If you are going to spew that old-time fire-and-brimstone religion, I am so out of here, Robbie. That is a cop-out. Don't try to hide behind your interpretation of the Bible. This is not about religious differences. This is about you being a fucking asshole and attacking my lover. Don't make this about me or God."

"How can you be fucking a man? Jesus, Dean—"

"With a little stretching and a lot of lube."

"Damn it, Dean!" Robbie spun around and punched a locker, denting the metal before he began to pace. "You don't know what it's like out there. They will find any reason to tear you down. You can't be with him!"

"Well, if you show me this mysterious 'they', then we can have a conversation and get this shit straight for once and for all."

Robbie glared.

"Well, since I don't see They and you are unwilling to talk—"

"It's the hair, isn't it?" Robbie sneered, suddenly going on the attack. "That's why you do it—why you like taking it up the ass. I should have known."

"It's not the hair, Robbie. This is just the way I am."

"That's why you hid it."

"I never hid anything."

"You are ashamed. You wanted us to guess, to help you out, so you grew your hair long. I should have known something was up when you started letting it grow out in high school. Or was it a trap to lure men in? It's as pretty as a girl's, I'll give you that—"

"It's not my fucking hair, Robbie. Look, I like pussy. I had my share in high school and college. But I love dick, Robbie. I love looking at it, I love touching it, sucking it, swallowing it, and I damn sure love fucking it. That is what makes me gay, not my fucking hair."

"It's a trap. You get good men fascinated by it and then you turn them."

"Like a vampire?" Dean had to laugh. "Like Night Of The Living Gays or some shit? Robbie," he drawled, "I thought you were smarter than that."

"You always thought you were better than everyone else—" Robbie shouted, advancing on Dean, who did not back down in the least. "Prancing around with your book smarts and your proper speech, and your fucking long hair—"

"You seem unduly interested in my hair, Robert. What's the matter? It turning you gay?"

"Fuck you!" Robbie roared in his face and Dean laughed. "Stop laughing at me you prick!" And that made Dean laugh harder.

He stopped laughing though, when a blow to the face sent him careening into a medical table near the lockers.

He shook off the pain and rose to his feet, one hand reaching out to touch the side of his mouth, noting the blood on his fingers before he turned to Robbie again.

The man was standing there, slack-jawed in disbelief, as he stared at Dean.

"Poor old Robbie Keton." Dean shook his head, noting that other than splitting his lip a little, Robbie's punch hadn't packed much of a wallop. "First everyone turns on you, abandons you, and it's never your fault." He looked down on the table and picked up a pair of scissors, snorting as Robbie began to look nervous. "It's the ball-busting dykes, and the geeks, and the people who take pride in themselves—and the gays. Let's not forget the fucking gays. And now it's my hair."

When he stepped forward, Robbie began to babble. "Dean—my God—I didn't mean to—"

"You never do." Dean shook his head. "You make racist comments because you didn't learn any better— which is a fucking lie. Half your team was black, Robbie. You call Coach a dyke because she is not interested in your fat ass. You call Dolton a spear-chucker because you attacked him and he kicked your monkey ass. And now I am gay because of my hair. I can't prove to you that you are wrong, you won't listen anyway, but I can do this."

Dean raised the scissors to his hair and began to cut. Hanks of long blond hair fell around his feet and he hacked and cut away.

"You think you are so tough because you were NFL. You think you know everything because you managed to play two seasons before you got ousted, probably because of your attitude."

"I didn't—"

"Shut up!" Dean roared, pointing the scissors in his direction. "You don't have leave to speak. A real man is talking and you will damn well listen."

Another handful of hair fell and he gathered the hair from his back in a loose grip and began to cut at that as well.

"You were so fucking smart, your second chance at starting over was just ruined because of your attitude way before you attacked. And now you are so smart that you just lost your last friend in this world."

Dean pulled the scissors away from his head and stared at the long strands that remained in his hand. Dolton was going to kill him, he decided as his temper began to ease and he stood there with unfamiliar air caressing the back of his neck.

"*So* fucking smart." He glared up at Robbie before he hurled his shorn hair in his face. "*So* smart that you know my fucking long hair made me gay. So there it is, buddy. And guess what? I still like dick. I guess Robbie Keton is *not as smart* as he thinks." He widened his eyes in feigned shock. "And I guess that means Robbie Keton was just plain wrong. And if he is wrong about this, think of how many other things he is wrong about." Then he narrowed his eyes as he glared at the remains of what used to be an okay man—not a good man or a great man, just an ordinary man. "I guess that just makes Robbie Keton an intolerant asshole."

"Dean…" Robbie's voice sounded broken as he stood there, Dean's blond hair sticking to his face and uniform.

"No." Dean shook his head. "You said what you had to say and I said what I had to. I guess this is the end."

"No," Robbie denied, taking a step forward. "I can help you…get you to some people who can—"

"Beat the gay out of me?" Dean snorted. "Not very likely, friend. But you know what they say—those who protest too much..."

Robbie's broken look turned to one of anger and again he reached for Dean, but Dean was ready. He easily sidestepped Robbie's clumsy attempt at grabbing him, spun around and ploughed his fist into his face. And unlike Robbie's sucker punch that had merely caught him off guard, his blow laid his ex-friend out flat.

"Don't touch me!" Dean bellowed, standing over the fallen man. "Don't you ever touch me! You don't have the right."

Arms around his chest prevented him from doing further damage and Dean spun around to see the angry visage of his lover looming over him.

Dolton stared at his lover for a brief moment, sadness in his eyes before he turned to look at the mess of Robbie, flat out in a pile of blond hair, blood once again tricking down from his nose.

"I think it's broken." He nodded to Robbie's face. The man was frozen, apparently too scared to move. Then Dolton looked Dean in the eyes. "You done here?"

"Yes, I am," Dean was proud to state. "Take me home and fuck me."

"Or I get a little kiss with your fist too?" he stated wryly, and Dean felt the tension in his body ease.

"You get that ass up for me and we can forgo the first kiss."

"Sounds like a plan."

Unburdened, the pair tuned and left, leaving behind nothing but bad memories and a new determination to make this thing between them work.

Chapter Nine

"My hair," Dolton moaned as he pulled Dean out of the Jacuzzi and sat him on a bench in the master bath off the master bedroom. "Did you have to cut off my hair?"

"It is *my* hair, love," Dean reminded his lover as the man pulled out the shaver he used to keep his own dome clean-shaven. "You just have to get over it."

"But it was perfect." Dolton began the process of balding his lover properly. "I think you should have hit him harder."

"I don't want to think about Robert Keton." Dean shook his now bald head as Dolton quickly whisked away any fallen strands of blond hair. He looked at himself in a mirror that his lover held for him and had to say that at least everyone could see his eyes now. "I tend to have a bit of a temper—"

"And you are a pushy bottom."

"Fuck you," Dean laughed.

"Just waiting on you." Dolton pointed out into the bedroom. "While you were showering and soaking, I set things up." His eyes turned molten as he stared down at him. "You promised me a lot of things, baby. And I want to see you keep your promises and deliver. There are condoms and lube in there and my favourite cuffs are waiting. Tie me up and fuck me."

"Oh yeah." Dean felt his cock leap to attention and smirked at his lover. "Do I have to tell you how to prepare—"

"Enema in the shower at the school," Dolton bragged, climbing onto the bed. "Ryan gave me a kit. I am as fresh as a daisy and ready to be fucked." He willingly stretched his arms out to the headboard and to the leather cuffs that hung there waiting. "Do your best."

With Dolton restrained on the bed, Dean easily spread his legs wide, exposing his tiny dark hole. Licking his lips, he stared at it until it twitched, then he looked up into his lover's golden eyes. "Hungry?"

"Peckish," Dolton answered, smirking at his lover. Although he was on the bottom and was giving up control nothing could take away the man's dominant presence. "So you gonna feed me or is this just a tease?"

In answer, Dean dived down and began tonguing his lovers' ass. He tasted darkly of musk, raw and masculine. It was a heady experience.

Dolton began to growl and thrust back against his face. Dean pulled back long enough to wet one finger deep in his mouth before he carefully slid it into his ass.

"Damn," he breathed as he felt the muscles clench around his fingers. "Are you doing that or has it just been a really long time since you got fucked?"

"It's been years." Dolton wigged and the vise around his finger eased off. "And I am controlling my muscles. Come on, give me more. I just wanted you to know in advance what it would feel like to sink balls deep inside me."

Dean groaned, cupping his balls to stem off a premature ejaculation. It had been a while since he had topped and he only hoped he could hold it together long enough for a good showing.

He looked over at his lover's heavy dick and leant forward to swallow it down his throat. He looked up at Dolton, his gaze challenging as the other man began to curse beneath his breath.

"We all have our skills," Dean popped his cock out of his mouth off long enough to say before he sucked him in deep again, making him arch his hips up and force that one finger in deeper.

Dean began a steady rhythm as he backed off and reached for the lube. He wet his fingers and pressed two into Dolton, keeping his dick sliding in and out of his throat. Two swiftly became three and Dolton was out of quips, his mouth hanging open and moans flowing freely. When he hit the man's prostate, his whole body stiffened, then melted into the mattress, leaving him open, wet and ready.

Dean abandoned his dick long enough to grab a condom and suit up before he was crawling up Dolton's body and slamming a harsh kiss onto his mouth.

"You are so pretty like that," he purred, watching as his lover's muscles bulged and shook under his inked skin. The many tattoos looked like they were dancing. Dean bent down and captured a nipple ring between his teeth, tugging at the ring of gold until Dolton whined and pressed his chest forward into the pain. Dean released it and licked away the slight pain before sucking the whole nipple in his mouth, flicking at the ring with his tongue.

"You do that so well," Dolton praised. "So good, baby. You gonna suck me again?"

"No," Dean backed off to say, one hand wrapping around Dolton's throbbing cock. "I'm just going to fuck you."

He looked down at the cherry-red angry head of his cock while he stroked the base. It was not hard as it was when he had been fucked through the mattress. Dolton was a willing bottom but it was obvious he preferred to top. It gave him an idea for later.

He spread his lover's legs wider and slid between them lifting Dolton's' hips and his ass to rest on his thighs.

He carefully parted his cheeks, drenched him in lube and pressed the head of his pink cock against the dark hole.

Dolton took a deep breath and relaxed, opening his body to his lover as Dean eased into the tight clench of Dolton's ass.

"Oh fuck," he moaned, sweat breaking out over his body as he sank deeper into Dolton. "So—so good—"

Dolton's face tightened for a moment then he blew out a deep breath as Dean began to sink in deeper.

"Damn," he gasped finally when Dean's balls were slapping against his ass. "My baby packin'—"

Dean would have laughed, but the tight stranglehold Dolton had on his cock had him counting backwards and mentally reciting the periodic table to prevent himself from blowing. Dolton was so tight, so hot and silky—and he was giving his ass up to Dean. He pulled out slowly and pushed back in hard when Dolton wrapped his legs around his waist and jerked him close.

"Fuck me!" he demanded. "I want to feel it burn."

Leaning over him, Dean took his mouth in a heated kiss while he began to plough his lover's ass.

Dolton took it so well, throwing his hips up and straining against the cuffs that held him in place. His head was rocking from side to side, his muscular body bouncing with each slam in, his eyes closed and a dreamy smile on his lips. He moaned softly with each withdrawal and tightened his leg around his waist on each thrust in. The sounds of their fucking filled the air and the scent of male heat was heavy in the room.

"Oh fuck — fuck — fuck —" Dean was muttering as he felt the tension in his body rise. His balls were filling, getting tight, his chest was heaving to take in air as he pounded his willing lover.

"Yeah —" Dolton was moaning louder and louder. "Yeah, baby. Make me feel it."

"Gonna come," Dean grunted after several moments of this. He rested his weight on his hands beside Dolton's head and moved harder, hovering over him, taking sucking kisses from his lips as he let his stomach caress the underside of his cock. "So hot and all mine," Dean purred, bent low and nipped at Dolton's neck. "So going to fucking come — so fucking hard —"

Then he could not form words as his blood roared in his ears and his whole body stiffened. His balls drew up and his cock swelled as it began to blast spurt after spurt of hot seed into the protective condom.

"Fuuuck!" he growled, his hips slamming in to get as deep as he could as he unloaded.

Beneath him Dolton was smirking, his eyes glowing in mirth even as his hard dick steadily leaked pre-cum between them.

"You are so beautiful when you come —" he began, but Dean rose up, gripped the base of the condom and pulled out.

The used rubber was tossed aside as Dean grabbed the lube and climbed to his knees.

He poured a generous amount onto Dolton's cock before sliding on a condom and lubing the barrier further.

"What—"

Before Dolton could ask, Dean was squatting over his lover's hard dick.

"Oh, fuck yeah." Dolton got with the programme pretty quickly, arching his hips and holding still.

Dean began to lower himself slowly, wincing as the soreness from before returned.

"Easy, baby," Dolton soothed. "You don't have to do this—"

"Shut up," Dean growled, his lover's voice breaking his concentration. Then he tuned the man out, focusing in on the thick dick stretching his ass to capacity.

The head popped in with a sharp burst of pain that was quickly forgotten as the broad head brushed against his prostate.

"Fuuck." He relaxed as he allowed gravity to assist in seating him. After a few moments, he opened his eyes when he bottomed out, seated fully, proudly, on his lover's dick.

"Let me loose, babe," Dolton asked. "I need to touch you."

"You need to sit there and take it."

He rose up, his whole body flexing under his lover's gaze before he dropped back down.

It burned, it hurt, and it felt so fucking good! He felt alive, unburdened and sex was just damn good fun when you were with someone like Dolton.

His lover was putting on a show, flexing his muscles, rocking his hips up to meet his thrusts as Dean took a ride on his dick.

"It hurts so good." Dean's head rolled back and he moaned, his body tightening as he adjusted his hips so that each stroke struck his prostate.

"F—fuck," Dolton stammered. "Ride me, baby. Ride that dick like you own it."

So Dean leaned over, his thighs spreading out wide giving Dolton an excellent view of his fat cock shiny with his seed, and his pink balls that contrasted so nicely with his darker skin. Then he was working his hips, one hand on Dolton's shoulder, the other on his stomach as he slammed himself back and forth.

There was no way he could come again, it was too soon, but he relished the feel of the hot throbbing cock deep inside him and the fact that he was giving his lover pleasure.

"Yeah, sir," he moaned, slipping easily back into a submissive mindset. "Fuck that ass. Tear it up. Fuck me!"

And Dolton was going wild, snorting and throwing his whole body up, tugging at the leather that held him in place. His body glistened with sweat, his tattoos a bright whirl as he writhed beneath him.

"Mmmm!"

Dolton was stiffening, his body arched up as his cock swelled to his fullest inside him. There was a pulsing as Dolton shouted his name, "Dean—God, baby!" and he could feel the extra heat as the condom was filled.

Dolton collapsed back onto the bed and Dean just sort of crumpled on top of him.

"My ass hurts," he commented after a moment, looking up into amused golden eyes.

"No one told you to ride me like a bronco buster, baby, not that I don't appreciate it."

"Hmm," he purred, rising up enough to take a few kisses before dropping his head on Dolton's chest.

"Let me free and I'll do good by you, baby," Dolton promised. "I swear."

"Bath and food?"

"If that is what you want. After all, you had a hard day, kicking ass and taking names — and cutting off my hair — "

"Yeah, yeah," Dean snorted, reaching up to undo the fastening that held Dolton's wrists bound.

His lover rested against him, pressing kisses to the top of his newly bald head.

"Does it look too bad?"

"Not like you have headquarters," Dolton joked. "You know, four separate humps to make a head — "

"Fuck you."

"You are beautiful, baby." Dolton wrapped him up tightly and gave him a squeeze before pushing him off his chest. "You are perfect no matter what you do to yourself. It is Dean Majors that I wanted in my bed and it is Dean Majors that I got. The hair was an unexpected bonus. It will grow back."

"Unless I like this look better — "

Dolton laughed, released him and rose to his feet. "I promised dinner and a bath. I'll get to work on that."

"Hmm," Dean purred, watching as his lover disposed of the condoms and did general maintenance before tugging on a robe.

"And if anyone asks, you can tell them that we are doing that lookalike thing to get over a hard part of our relationship. Your ass wants a vacation and my dick just can't let go."

"Fuck you," Dean laughed, snuggling into the warm blankets.

"Already did," Dolton returned. "And I got you to watch my back if anyone says anything. When they find out what a wicked left you have — "

Dean tuned out his lover's joking and let himself doze.

He might have lost a friend, but he had gained a lover who would defend him and stand by him. He had a stable relationship they were still exploring and it looked like his life was falling into place. Not too bad of a trade-off.

As he relaxed, he could hear Dolton puttering around him singing...sounding like his future. He closed his eyes and went to sleep.

Epilogue

The next time they showed up to practise sporting identical do's the Griffins, one of the toughest teams in the league, just shrugged it off without too much comment. Looked like the grid iron had borne another relationship and like any relationship forged in steel, and hardened in the fires of dedication and perseverance, it appeared that this one was going to last.

In the stands the spectators cheered, on the field the defensive line were flattening everything that threatened their quarterback, and on the sidelines, a woman dressed in scarlet red shoes took a look at her team in green and black and smiled in contentment.

About the Authors

Cheryl Dragon

A lover of unusual things, Cheryl Dragon enjoys writing unique stories with sinfully hot erotic romance. Her two favourite settings are Las Vegas and New Orleans…where anything can happen! Cheryl lives in the Chicagoland area with her deaf albino cat. By day she analyses numbers for a division of a large international conglomerate, which leaves the creative juices free for her erotic romance novels.

Megan Slayer

When she's not writing the stories in her head, Megan Slayer can be found luxuriating in her hot tub with her two vampire Cabana boys, Luke and Jeremy. She has the tendency to run a tad too far with her muse, so she has to hide in the head of her alter ego, but the boys don't seem to mind.

When she's not obsessing over her whip collection, she can be found picking up her kidlet from school.

She enjoys writing in all genres, but writing about men in love suits her fancy best.

Stephanie Burke

Have You Been Flashed?

It's the question Stephanie Burke is asking.

Stephanie is a multi published multi award-winning wife and mother of two whose unparalleled imagination causes her no end of trouble.

From sex shifting shape-shifting dragons to under sea worlds, up to sexually confused elemental fey and homo erotic mysteries, all the way to pastel challenged urban sprites, Stephanie has done it all, and hopes to do more.

Stephanie an Orator on her favourite subject of writing and world building, a sometimes teacher when you feed her enough coffee and donuts, an anime nut, a costumer, and a frequent guest of various sci-fi and writing cons where she can be found leading panel discussions or researching more and varied legends and theories to improve her writing skills.

Stephanie is known for her love of the outrageous, strong female characters, believable worlds, male characters filled with depth, and interracial that make the reader sit up and take notice.

All of the above authors love to hear from readers. You can find their contact information, website details and author profile pages at http://www.totallybound.com.

Totally Bound Publishing

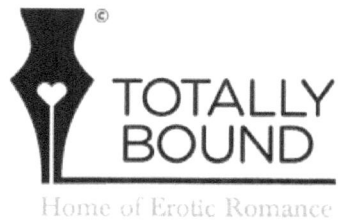

www.ingramcontent.com/pod-product-compliance
Lightning Source LLC
Chambersburg PA
CBHW032027240626

47154CB00003B/816